HAEMATOLOGY
FOR THE MRCP

HAEMATOLOGY FOR THE MRCP

DAVID W. GALVANI

MD, MRCP, MRCPath
Consultant Haematologist
Department of Haematology
Arrowe Park Hospital, Upton, Wirral
Merseyside

WB SAUNDERS COMPANY LTD

LONDON   PHILADELPHIA   TORONTO
SYDNEY   TOKYO

W. B. Saunders
Company Ltd

24–28 Oval Road
London NW1 7DX, UK

The Curtis Center
Independence Square West
Philadelphia, PA 19106-3399
USA

Harcourt Brace & Company
55 Horner Avenue
Toronto, Ontario M8Z 4X6
Canada

Harcourt Brace & Company
Australia
30–52 Smidmore Street
Marrickville, NSW 2204
Australia

Harcourt Brace & Company
Japan Inc.
Ichibancho Central Building
22–1 Ichibancho
Chiyoda-ku, Tokyo 102, Japan

© 1995 W. B. Saunders Company Ltd

A catalogue record for this book is available from the
British Library

ISBN 0–7020–1883–X

This book is printed on acid-free paper

Typeset by Selwood Systems, Midsomer Norton and printed
and bound in Great Britain by Mackays of Chatham PLC

CONTENTS

for Jill, Tim and Marco

PREFACE

The MRCP examination requires a broad breadth of reading, but
also considerable clinical experience. This can make preparation
for this exam difficult and people worry about unusual problems
that they have not read about or experienced. It is very sensible,
therefore, to prepare for the examination by performing practice
examinations. This book aims to cover the main areas that crop
up in the exam such as megaloblastic anaemia and leukaemias etc,
but in addition it also aims to inform and educate about
conditions which are less common but which can appear in the
MRCP in various guises.

Pattern recognition plays a large part in this type of exam, so
try to assimilate all the data that you are given and think
laterally, information is not usually given in order to mislead.
Sometimes it is this wealth of information which causes
confusion and difficulty, especially for those people with less
experience in dealing with the complexities of clinical life. If the
answer is obvious, state it clearly and do not couch it in
unnecessary waffle. If the answer is less clear describe the
abnormalities and at least give some sort of sensible differential
diagnosis in a clear fashion. Do not forget, examiners hate
meandering waffle.

Most of these questions have been tried and tested on MRCP
candidates over the last year and they tell me that the majority
are fair and reasonable. If you come across a question or
condition with which you are unfamiliar, do not despair but use
it as an opportunity to learn something new. I find that MRCP
candidates make the mistake of re-reading what they know
instead of taking the more difficult option of going out and
learning new facts about conditions with which they are
unfamiliar. Do not forget, you may get an unusual or obscure
long case and it is as well to at least know something about it.
Good luck.

DAVID GALVANI

ABBREVIATIONS

ACD	anaemia of chronic disease
AIDS	acquired immune deficiency syndrome
ALG	antilymphocyte globulin
Alk Phos	alkaline phosphatase
ALL	acute lymphoblastic leukaemia
ALT	alanine transferase
AML	acute myeloid leukaemia
ANF	antinuclear factor
APS	antiphospholipid syndrome
APTT	activated partial thromboplastin time (= KCTT)
ARDS	acute respiratory distress syndrome
AST	aspartate transferase
ATIII	antithrombin III
ATRA	all-*trans*-retinoic acid
AZT	azidothymidine
BMT	bone marrow transplantation
BP	blood pressure
CGL	chronic granulocytic leukaemia
CLL	chronic lymphocytic leukaemia
CML	chronic myeloid leukaemia
CMV	cytomegalovirus
CNS	central nervous system
CSF	colony-stimulating factor
CXR	chest X-ray
DAF	decay-accelerating factor
DDAVP	desamino D-arginyl vasopressin
DEB	diepoxybutane
DIC	disseminated intravascular coagulation
DRVVT	dilute Russell's viper venom test
DVT	deep venous thrombosis
EBV	Epstein–Barr virus
ECG	electrocardiography
ELISA	enzyme-linked immunosorbent assay

ESR	erythrocyte sedimentation rate
FA	Fanconi's anaemia
FBC	full blood count
FFP	fresh frozen plasma
FMLP	f-met-leu-phe
G6PD	glucose-6-phosphate dehydrogenase
G-CSF	granulocyte colony-stimulating factor
GGT	gamma glutamyl transferase
GIT	gastrointestinal tract
GM-CSF	granulocyte-macrophage colony-stimulating factor
GVHD	graft versus host disease
Hb	haemoglobin
HBsAg	hepatitis B surface antigen
HCL	hairy cell leukaemia
HCV	hepatitis C
HD	Hodgkin's disease
HIV	human immunodeficiency virus
HLA	human leukocyte antigen
HS	hereditary spherocytosis
HUS	haemolytic–uraemic syndrome
ITP	idiopathic (immune) thrombocytopenia
IFN	interferon
Ig	immunoglobulin
IL	interleukin
IVIG	intravenous immunoglobulin
KCCT	kaolin cephalin clotting time (=APTT)
LAP	leukocyte alkaline transferase
LGL	large granular lymphocytes
MAHA	microangiopathic haemolytic anaemia
MCH	mean corpuscular haemoglobin
MCHC	mean corpuscular haemoglobin concentration
MCV	mean corpuscular volume
MDS	myelodysplastic states
MF	myelofibrosis
MGUS	monoclonal gammopathy of uncertain significance
MI	myocardial infarction
NHL	non-Hodgkin's lymphoma

NK	natural killer (cells)
NMR	nuclear magnetic resonance
NSAID	non-steroidal anti-inflammatory drug
PAI-1	plasminogen activator inhibitor-1
PCP	*Pneumocystis carinii* pneumonia
P_{CO_2}	partial pressure of CO_2
PCV	packed cell volume
PET	pre-eclamptic toxaemia
Pl IgG	platelet-associated immunoglobulin G
PML	promyelocytic leukaemia
PNH	paroxysmal nocturnal haemoglobinuria
P_{O_2}	partial pressure of O_2
PPP	primary proliferative polycythaemia
PT	prothrombin time
PTP	post-transfusion purpura
RAR	retinoic acid receptor
RBC	red blood cell
RCC	red cell count
RCM	red cell mass
RDW	red cell distribution width
RiCof	ristocetin cofactor
SABE	subacute bacterial endocarditis
SLE	systemic lupus erythematosis
TB	tuberculosis
TIBC	total iron-binding capacity
TSH	thyroid-stimulating hormone
TT	thrombin time
TTP	thrombotic thrombocytopenic purpura
UMN	upper motor neurone
vWD	von Willebrand's disease
vWF	von Willebrand's factor
vWFAg	von Willebrand's factor antigen
WCC	white cell count
ZPP	zinc protoporphyrin

CASE HISTORIES

CASE HISTORIES
QUESTIONS

1. A 43-year-old Black midwife had attended the hypertension clinic for 3 years. Her BP had been 136/85 on 100 mg atenolol daily. Regular haematological and biochemical screening had been normal. Urinalysis had detected protein intermittently. She had had 2 full-term normal deliveries and was heterozygous for Hb S. She was a non-smoker and drank alcohol rarely. Her mother died of tuberculosis.

At her follow-up appointment she presented with a 6-week history of lethargy, and pain in her lower back for 3 weeks. On examination there were no specific findings; BP 145/90. Urinalysis: protein +.
Haematology: Hb 9.6 g/dl, MCV 83 fl, platelets $122 \times 10^9/l$, WCC $3.6 \times 10^9/l$ (neutrophils 1.2, lymphocytes 2.1).
ESR 78 mm/h, serum electrophoresis showed a κ light-chain monoclonal paraprotein, IgG 7.8 g/l, IgA 1.2 g/l, IgM 0.5 g/l (normal ranges: IgG 5–14 g/l, IgA 1–4 g/l, IgM 0.5–2.0 g/l).
Biochemistry: serium calcium 2.76 mmol/l, albumin 37 g/l, globulin 28 g/l, urea 14 mmol/l, creatinine 256 μmol/l.
Autoantibody screen: normal.
Skeletal survey demonstrated areas of osteoporosis.
Marrow aspirate: normal.

(a) What is the most likely diagnosis?
(b) How can this be confirmed?
(c) What are the prognostic implications?

2. A 34-year-old housewife had presented with ITP 3 years ago. She responded initially to a course of prednisolone but relapsed on 10 mg/day. Her platelet count proved resistant to increasing the dose of prednisolone and a splenectomy

was performed. The platelet count had been stable at around 110 to 120 × 10⁹/l since that time. She had had 1 full-term normal delivery. There was no family history of note. She was a non-smoker and did not drink alcohol. She recently presented to her general practitioner with a left DVT and vague discomfort in her anterior chest. Venography confirmed a DVT within the left femoral vein, and the CXR was normal. She was admitted for anticoagulation and was found to have a soft systolic murmur. Ultrasound of the abdomen revealed no abdominal pathology or pregnancy. Hb 10.6 g/dl, platelets 132 × 10⁹/l, WCC 6.4 × 10⁹/l (neutrophils 1.5, lymphocytes 4.6). Film: polychromasia, target cells, Howell-Jolly bodies, some spherocytes. Coombs' test positive (for IgG). Prior to anticoagulation: PT 14 s (control 15 s), KCCT 35 s (control 29 s), TT 10 s (control 9 s).

(a) What is the most likely diagnosis and how would you confirm this?
(b) What complications have occurred?
(c) How would you manage and monitor anticoagulation?

3. A 27-year-old Chinese woman was proving large for dates during the 24th week of her second pregnancy. She had a BP of 140/95, mild pedal oedema, and protein and glucose on urinalysis. Ultrasound revealed a large fetus with enlarged liver and spleen, ascites and pleural effusions. The biparietal diameter was in keeping with the 24th week of pregnancy. Biochemistry: fasting plasma glucose 6.5 mmol/l. Serum albumin 38 g/l, globulin 25 g/l, urea 8 mmol/l, creatinine 122 μmol/l, bilirubin 16 μmol/l, AST 25 U/l, ALT 20 U/l. Haematology: Hb 10.3 g/dl, MCV 69 fl, platelets 188 × 10⁹/l, WCC 9.8 × 10⁹/l (normal differential). Blood film: microcytic with target cells. Blood group O, Rhesus positive (*CDE/cde* genotype). Iron studies proved normal, therefore Hb electrophoresis was performed: Hb A 97%, Hb A₂ 2.5% (normal 2.2–3.3), Hb F < 1%, Hb S not detected. She had had 1 previous normal pregnancy. She was a non-

smoker and did not drink alcohol. There was no family history of note.

(a) What do you suspect is the haematological diagnosis in the mother and fetus?
(b) How can this be confirmed?
(c) Why do you need to see the father of the child?

4. A 35-year-old man complained of increasing dyspnoea of effort with intermittent fever over the previous 2 weeks. He had lost 4 kg in the previous month. On examination he was pale, had non-tender bilateral cervical lymphadenopathy (glands 1.5 cm diameter), splenomegaly (8 cm), hepatomegaly (4 cm), reduced air entry and dullness in the right upper lobe with stony dullness at the left base.
FBC: Hb 9.5 g/dl, MCV 84 fl, platelets 527×10^9/l, WCC 6.2×10^9/l (neutrophils 3.4, lymphocytes 2.0, eosinophils 0.6). Film: Polychromasia, mild eosinophilia. Coombs' test positive (for IgG).
Biochemistry: serum albumin 40 g/l, globulin 30 g/l, ALT 84 U/l, AST 122 U/l, Alk Phos 140 U/l, calcium 2.6 mmol/l, urea 5.4 mmol/l, creatinine 102 μmol/l.
Bone marrow: normal.
CXR: Shadowing right upper lobe, coarse infiltrative changes both lungs, moderate hilar lymphadenopathy, small left pleural effusion.
He was a non-smoker and drank 10 units of alcohol per week (on average). He lived with his wife and 3 children. He was a bank clerk and had not been abroad recently.

(a) What is the most likely diagnosis, and what definitive investigation is indicated?
(b) Give 2 other differential diagnoses with appropriate investigations.

5. A 24-year-old housewife presented to her general practitioner with progressive cough and dyspnoea. A weeks' course of erythromycin produced no benefit and she was referred to hospital. On examination she had a small conjunctival haemorrhage, was pale, not cyanosed and had no lymphadenopathy. She had signs of consolidation at the

left base; a CXR confirmed left lower lobe pneumonia.
Sputum grew pneumococcus. Full blood count revealed Hb
6.7 g/dl, MCV 103 fl, platelets $5 \times 10^9/l$, WCC $2.9 \times 10^9/l$
(neutrophils 0.2, lymphocytes 2.5, eosinophils 0.1,
monocytes 0.1 – blood film confirmed this differential). PT
14 s (control 15 s), APTT 38 s (control 37 s). Serum urea 5.6
mmol/l, creatinine 79 µmol/l, calcium 2.54 mmol/l,
bilirubin 17 µmol/l, AST 21 U/l, ALT 26 U/l. Bone marrow
aspirate was dry; trephine revealed aplasia with less than
10% normal cellularity and no clumps of cancer cells.
She was given filtered CMV-negative blood products as
support plus intravenous benzylpenicillin. A 5-day course
of horse antilymphocyte globulin (ALG) was administered
(plus steroid cover). Although her chest infection improved,
her pancytopenia failed to improve significantly in the next
4–6 weeks and she remained on blood product support.
Both her siblings proved incompatible for transplantation.
In an effort to boost her neutrophil count, a 7-day course of
G-CSF was given. Her WCC rose to $4.6 \times 10^9/l$ (neutrophils
0.4, lymphocytes 2.8, monocytes 0.2, myeloblasts 1.2). A
repeat marrow aspirate was performed.

(a) What further significant features would you elicit from
this history?
(b) What is the most likely haematological diagnosis?
(c) What are the toxicities of antilymphocyte globulin, and
why is steroid cover given?

6. A 53-year-old woman was admitted with confusion and an
apparent left-sided transient ischaemic attack. She had been
found to be hypertensive 10 years ago, following a 'small
stroke', and had been commenced on methyldopa, which
had controlled her BP at around 145/90. Her admission
haematology revealed Hb 11.1 g/dl, MCV 83 fl, platelets 65
$\times 10^9/l$, WCC $11.7 \times 10^9/l$ (neutrophils 9.5, lymphocytes
2.2). PT 15 s (control 14 s), APTT 38 s (control 37 s). Urea
8.6 mmol/l, creatinine 168 µmol/l. CXR: normal. ECG
showed sinus rhythm with mild left heart hypertrophy and
no evidence of infarction.
The following morning, examination revealed an obese

woman with a pyrexia of 38°C, normal heart sounds and sinus rhythm; left-sided upper motor neurone (UMN) signs had resolved; the abdomen was slightly distended but no organomegaly or guarding was elicited. Information from her general practitioner and her elderly sister revealed that she may have had a urinary infection 2 weeks earlier, that she rarely ventured out and that she had not experienced angina or claudication to their knowledge. Repeat haematology revealed Hb 10.4 g/dl, platelets 23×10^9/l, WCC 13.7×10^9/l (neutrophils 11.2, lymphocytes 2.3), PT 16 s (control 14 s), APTT 40 s (control 37 s). Serum sodium 139 mmol/l, potassium 4.6 mmol/l, calcium 2.63 mmol/l, urea 10.2 mmol/l, creatinine 182 μmol/l, albumin 42 g/l, globulin 27 g/l. The blood film confirmed neutrophilia and thrombocytopenia, and revealed schistocytes.
Her general condition deteriorated with confusion and fever, and she was commenced on antibiotics.

(a) What is the most likely cause of her thrombocytopenia?
(b) Give a differential diagnosis.
(c) What management would you advise?

7. A 28-year-old woman booked into antenatal clinic at 11 weeks with her first pregnancy. She volunteered that she did not have a regular sexual partner and used the contraceptive pill intermittently. She worked as a clerk. There was no past medical history or drug history of note. Examination revealed a BP of 110/80, no oedema, and uterine enlargement that was compatible with 11 weeks' gestation. Initial investigations revealed Hb 11.6 g/dl, MCV 90 fl, platelets 96×10^9/l, WCC 10.5×10^9/1 (neutrophils 8.2, lymphocytes 2.1). Blood group O, Rhesus positive (*CDe/CDe* genotype), no detectable red cell antibodies. Urinalysis: protein +, sugar negative, no bacterial growth. No further action was taken at this point.
At 20 weeks' gestation, the woman had no major symptoms of note. BP was 130/80; no oedema or jaundice was detected; weight gain was appropriate, fundus compatible with 20 weeks' gestation. Urinalysis: protein +, sugar +, no bacterial growth. Repeat blood count showed Hb 11.3 g/dl,

platelets 36×10^9/l, WCC 12.5×10^9/l (neutrophils 9.8, lymphocytes 2.4). Serum urea 3.6 mmol/l, creatinine 86 μmol/l, bilirubin 11 μmol/l, AST 17 U/l, glutamyl transferase (GGT) 26 U/l, Alk Phos 89 U/l.

(a) What further tests are now indicated?
(b) What is the most likely diagnosis?
(c) Give a differential diagnosis of thrombocytopenia in pregnancy.
(d) What management would you recommend?

8. A 29-year-old woman with known homozygous sickle cell disease had had several sickle crises throughout her life. She had developed a chronic leg ulcer on the left ankle. She lived with her husband, had no children and did not smoke or drink. She took penicillin prophylactically. She had 1 brother who also had sickle cell disease.
She was admitted with an 18-hour history of severe pain in her left elbow and extreme lethargy. On examination she was pale and icteric. Pulse 120/min, BP 90/70, respirations 30/min. There was a soft systolic murmur at the apex. Chest expansion was full with no added sounds. Her abdomen was swollen, with 10 cm hepatomegaly but no splenomegaly, her left elbow was slightly swollen and stiff. There were no neurological signs.
Haematology: Hb 4.6 g/dl, MCV 82 fl, platelets 869×10^9/l, WCC 12.6×10^9/l (neutrophils 10.2, lymphocytes 2.1). PT 18 s (control 16 s), APTT 39 s (control 36 s), fibrinogen 2.3 g/l. Serological screening revealed antibodies to Duffy and Kell red cell antigens.
Biochemistry: serum sodium 137 mmol/l, potassium 4.2 mmol/l, urea 6.3 mmol/l, creatinine 99 μmol/l, bilirubin 78 μmol/l (unconjugated 48 μmol/l), AST 148 U/l, Alk Phos 385 U/l, GGT 93 U/l, albumin 41 g/l, globulin 30 g/l.
pH 7.43, $P\text{O}_2$ 10.5 kPa, $P\text{CO}_2$ 3.5 kPa, bicarbonate 25 mmol/l. CXR: clear.

(a) What is the most likely diagnosis?
(b) What management would you recommend?
(c) What are the practical implications of the red cell antibodies?

9. A 7-year-old boy presented to his general practitioner with recurrent gum bleeding following brushing his teeth. His parents commented that he had been more lethargic lately, and had been less inclined to join in games. They also commented that he had been struggling to keep up with his school work.
On examination he was small for his age with an 'elfin' appearance. He had 3 café au lait spots and his thumbs appeared abnormal.
Biochemistry: serum sodium 143 mmol/l, potassium 4.6 mmol/l, bicarbonate 29 mmol/l, urea 8.6 mmol/l and creatinine 210 μmol/l.
Haematology: Hb 8.6 g/dl, platelets 31×10^9/l, WCC 6.3×10^9/l (neutrophils 2.1, lymphocytes 2.3, blasts 2.0).
Bone marrow aspirate was hypocellular with dysplastic features in all cell lines; 50% of nucleated cells were blasts, and these were Sudan black positive. Bone trephine was also hypocellular and contained several groups of large nucleolated cells.

(a) What is the most likely diagnosis?
(b) Name the definitive test.
(c) What counselling would you offer the family?

10. A 33-year-old man was admitted with a definite anterior myocardial infarction. Examination revealed: pulse 100/min (sinus rhythm), BP 140/90, minimal cardiac failure, no evidence of coarctation, heart sounds normal, moderately overweight.
Admission results revealed Hb 20.3 g/dl, packed cell volume (PCV) 0.61, MCV 82 fl, WCC 12.1×10^9/l (neutrophils 8.7, lymphocytes 2.4), platelets 442×10^9/l.
Serum sodium 139 mmol/l, potassium 3.8 mmol/l, urea 9.5 mmol/l, creatinine 154 μmol/l. Urinalysis: protein ++, sugar negative.
A haematological opinion was sought and 2 units of blood were transfused over the course of 3 days. He made a good recovery and during convalescence his red cell mass was measured as 30 ml/kg (normal 25–35), plasma volume 29 ml/kg (normal 40–50). A diagnosis of

'pseudopolycythaemia' was made. Urine protein was measured as 6.8 g/day, creatinine clearance was 80 ml/min. Hypertension had been diagnosed 1 year previously when he presented with a left DVT. He had received a 3 month course of warfarin and his BP was well controlled on atenolol and nifedipine. He was a British Telecom engineer, did not smoke and consumed 10 units of alcohol per week.

(a) Give the most likely cause of his polycythaemia, and discuss the red cell mass and plasma volume results.
(b) Give 2 further investigations that you think are essential to provide an accurate diagnosis.
(c) What further haematological investigations are indicated?

11. A 34-year-old man presented to his general practitioner with profound fatigue. His blood count revealed: Hb 6.7 g/dl, MCV 86 fl, MCHC 37 g/dl, reticulocytes 0.5%, platelets 257×10^9/l, WCC 5.3×10^9/l (neutrophils 2.5). He had recently had a 'flu-like' illness, which he had caught from his wife. Bone marrow revealed normal myelopoiesis and megakaryocytes, but erythropoiesis was markedly suppressed.
His childhood was healthy and he had had a cholecystectomy at the age of 30 years. He worked as a garage mechanic, was a non-smoker and drank 15 units of alcohol per week. He has 1 brother and no children.

(a) What is the most likely diagnosis?
(b) How would you confirm this?
(c) What are the other complications of this disease?

12. A 60-year-old man was admitted with vesicobullous eruptions upon an erythemic base, these were present mainly over the trunk and upper arms. Lesions were 0.5–2.0 cm in diameter and were mainly flaccid in nature, Nikolsky's sign was positive. There were also several denuded areas over his back. He had several ulcers on his lips and mouth. There was a tense blister over his left palm and the occasional target lesion. Apart from the skin lesions he did not feel particularly unwell and was afebrile. He had

a few enlarged lymph nodes in both cervical regions and splenomegaly of 4 cm.

Haematology: Hb 9.4 g/dl, MCV 107 fl, platelets 167 × 10^9/l, WCC 20.1 × 10^9/l (neutrophils 5.6, lymphocytes 14.3). Blood film showed some anisocytosis and poikilocytosis but no polychromasia; mature lymphocytes were increased and occasional smear cells were seen.

Biochemistry: serum albumin 36 g/l, globulin 36 g/l, IgG 20 g/l, IgA 1.3 g/l, IgM 0.5 g/l. Immune fixation revealed an IgG κ band. Serum calcium 2.45 mmol/l, urea 7.4 mmol/l, creatinine 132 μmol/l.

CXR: normal.

(a) What is the haematological diagnosis and what complication(s) have developed?
(b) What is the dermatological diagnosis?
(c) How can the dermatological diagnosis be confirmed accurately?

13. A 38-year-old man was referred to the Haematology Clinic for investigation. He had always been an active squash player and runner, but had become increasingly fatigued with exercise over the last few months. He enjoyed good health, although as a young adult he had had three episodes of bone pain in his legs, associated with fever. He had received treatment for presumed osteomyelitis and had made a good recovery. Within the previous year he had been told by an orthopaedic surgeon that he was developing osteoarthrosis in both knees.

He enjoyed his work as an engineer in the family company, which had been established by his father, who was a Polish émigré. He was a non-smoker and drank 10 units of alcohol per week. He took no medication. He had travelled only in Northern Europe.

He had a healthy brother and healthy sister. He had 1 daughter but she died following progressive spasticity at 3 months of age; a definite diagnosis was never made. He also had a first cousin back in Poland who had been given a diagnosis of motor neurone disease.

On examination he was a fit man of average build. He had

hepatomegaly (3 cm), splenomegaly (6 cm) but no lymphadenopathy. There were no stigmata of liver disease. Neurological examination was normal. Both knees were slightly swollen and tender to palpation, but no restriction of movement was found.
Haematology: Hb 11.2 g/dl, MCV 84 fl, platelets 103 × 10⁹/l, WCC 5.3 × 10⁹/l (neutrophils 1.9, lymphocytes 3.1).
Blood film and Hb electrophoresis: normal.
Biochemistry: serum sodium 139 mmol/l, potassium 3.9 mmol/l, bicarbonate 28 mmol/l, chloride 99 mmol/l, urea 6.1 mmol/l, creatinine 112 μmol/l, calcium 2.5 mmol/l, albumin 40 g/l, globulin 27 g/l, AST 83 U/l, ALT 74 U/l, Alk Phos 266 U/l.
Autoantibody screen: negative.
Immune electrophoresis: normal.
CT scan of chest and abdomen showed no lymphadenopathy but confirmed the hepatosplenomegaly.

(a) What is the most likely diagnosis?
(b) Give 2 ways of confirming this.

14. A 40-year-old woman had been investigated for a Coombs'-positive anaemia 12 months ago. At that time no underlying pathology had been detected, and her anaemia had responded very well to a 6-week course of steroid therapy. She returned to her doctor because she had developed a cough and mild dysphagia. She had also lost a stone in weight, and had noticed intermittent fevers and troublesome generalized pruritis. She was found to be pale with cervical and axillary lymphadenopathy, and spelomegaly of 6 cm.
Haematological investigations revealed Hb 9.5 g/dl, MCV 96 fl, platelets 263 × 10⁹/l, WCC 8.8 × 10⁹/l (neutrophils 6.4, lymphocytes 1.9, eosinophils 0.4). Blood film showed polychromasia and spherocytes. Coombs' test positive. Reticulocytes 194 × 10⁹/l. Bone marrow aspirate was very cellular with erythroid hyperplasia.
Biochemistry: serum albumin 43 g/l, globulin 42 g/l with a polyclonal increase in all immunoglobulin fractions. Serum calcium 2.5 mmol/l, sodium 137 mmol/l, potassium 6.4

mmol/l, bicarbonate 19 mmol/l, urea 20.3 mmol/l, creatinine 673 µmol/l.
Antinuclear factor weakly positive. A cryoglobulin was detected.
CXR revealed mediastinal and hilar lymphadenopathy but no pulmonary pathology. Renal ultrasound showed slightly enlarged kidneys with dilatation of both calyces.

(a) What is the most likely diagnosis and what complications have occurred?
(b) How should the diagnosis be confirmed?

15. A 20-year-old male student went on holiday with his parents to the Gambia. He did not take regular malaria prophylaxis because it made him nauseous. Several days after returning home he developed fever and malaise, and noticed that his urine was red. He was admitted to hospital and a diagnosis of malaria was confirmed (*Plasmodium ovale*). On admission he was fully alert and oriented. He was pale and mildly icteric, he had 4 cm splenomegaly but no lymphadenopathy, and his temperature was 39°C. Urinalysis revealed blood and protein but no sugar; microscopy showed few intact red cells and no organisms, culture was also negative. FBC showed Hb 8.4 g/dl, MCV 95 fl, platelets 145 × 10⁹/l, WCC 16.4 × 10⁹/l (neutrophils 14.3, lymphocytes 2.0). Reticulocytes 210 × 10⁹/l, Blood film showed a few bite cells and spherocytes, polychromasia and intracellular parasites. Bilirubin 48 µmol/l, urea 6.4 mmol/l, creatinine 112 µmol/l.
He was commenced on chloroquine and primaquine and his temperature fell to 37°C. However, his urine remained red and urine output fell to 300 ml/day. Plasma urea and creatinine began rising rapidly over the next 2 days and Hb fell to 5.6 g/dl, MCV 100 fl, platelets 135 × 10⁹/l, WCC 14.3 × 10⁹/l (neutrophils 12.6, lymphocytes 1.7). Reticulocytes 250 × 10⁹/l. Bilirubin 92 µmol/l, ALT 36 U/l, Alk Phos 127 U/l.
He was single, a non-smoker, did not drink alcohol and was on no regular medication. He was a first-generation Egyptian. He had no history of major illnesses. There was no family history of note, and he was the only child.

(a) What is the diagnosis?
(b) How can this be confirmed?
(c) What management would you recommend?

16. A 49-year-old man presented with a 1-month history of intermittent colicky upper abdominal pain, anorexia and nausea. He had no significant diarrhoea, vomiting or weight loss. He had had similar but less severe episodes in the 6 months preceding his presentation and had also complained of severe headaches intermittently for 3 months.

He was an engineer and did not smoke. He consumed approximately 10 units of alcohol per week (never heavier than this). He had a normal diet of meat and vegetables and does not partake of any unusual foods. He had travelled to the east coast of America and in Germany, but not in the tropics. He was on no regular medication. His wife and 2 children are completely well.

The patient enjoyed good health and was reasonably fit although he had had a DVT in his right leg when he was 47 years old; he had received warfarin for 3 months following this episode.

On examination he was pale and icteric with a temperature of 37.2°C. He was fully orientated with no evidence of a liver flap or stigmata of chronic liver disease. There was hepatomegaly of 6 cm, a splenic tip and ascites, but no palpable lymphadenopathy.

Haematology: Hb 9.6 g/dl, MCV 96, platelets 96×10^9/l, WCC 4.3×10^9/l (neutrophils 1.5, lymphocytes 2.5). Blood film showed normochromic normocytic anaemia. PT 28 s (control 15 s), APTT 34 s (control 32 s), TT 10 s (control 10 s), fibrinogen 2.4 g/l.

Biochemistry: serum sodium 138 mmol/l, potassium 4.3 mmol/l, urea 5.7 mmol/l, creatinine 124 μmol/l, calcium 2.5 mmol/l, albumin 30 g/l, globulin 21 g/l, bilirubin 165 μmol/l, AST 126 U/l, ALT 232 U/l, GGT 143 U/l and Alk Phos 372 U/l.

Autoantibody screen: negative.

Virology screen: negative (including hepatitis A, B and C). There was no evidence of leptospirosis or brucella. Blood cultures were negative.

CXR: normal. Ultrasound examination confirmed an enlarged liver and spleen with ascites, but there were no gallstones or focal lesions within the liver. Isotope liver scan showed reduced but patchy uptake; however, the caudate lobe was enlarged and spared.
Bone marrow aspirate: dry. Marrow biopsy showed hypoplasia.

   (a) What is the most likely hepatological diagnosis and how can this be confirmed?
   (b) What is the most likely haematological diagnosis and how can this be confirmed?
   (c) What initial management would you recommend?

17. A 52-year-old woman with a 5-year history of rheumatoid arthritis had had several flare-ups of her disease but had been controlled mainly by NSAIDs. Although hand radiographs had demonstrated a few erosions, she had not required gold or penicillamine. At her most recent clinic visit she told her physician that she had had several chest infections over the course of the previous 6 months, and that she was feeling generally weaker, although her arthritis was reasonably quiet.
She was a housewife. She smoked 10 cigarettes per day but has abstained from alcohol for 10 years having been warned by her general practitioner that her consumption of 40 units per week was in danger of damaging her liver. She had had 2 normal pregnancies. She took only diclofenac sodium (Voltarol). She had never travelled abroad. There is no family history of note.
On examination she had swelling of the metacarpophalangeal joints with minimal ulnar deviation, and her wrist joints were slightly swollen but not warm. Range of movement was almost full in these joints, but the right shoulder had reduced extension and internal rotation. She had 10 cm splenomegaly but no hepatomegaly, stigmata of chronic liver disease or ascites. No lymphadenopathy was detected.
Haematology: Hb 10.7 g/dl, MCV 87 fl, platelets 136 × 10^9/l, WCC 6.7 × 10^9/l (neutrophils 0.4, lymphocytes 6.2).

Blood film showed normochromic features with activated lymphocytes.
Biochemistry: serum electrolytes normal, urea 6.2 mmol/l, creatinine 93 µmol/l, calcium 2.24 mmol/l, albumin 40 g/l, globulin 30 g/l, bilirubin 18 µmol/l, Alk Phos 120 U/l, ALT 30 U/l, GGT 45 U/l.
Rheumatoid factor 1/512, antinuclear factor (ANF) negative, antineutrophil antibodies positive.

(a) Give a differential diagnosis.
(b) What further haematological investigations are necessary?
(c) What management would you recommend?

18. A 52-year-old man presented with tiredness and increasing difficulty coping with his job in November 1992. At that time his general practitioner found that his Hb was 8.6 g/dl, MCV 82 fl, platelets 196 × 10⁹/l, WCC 5.3 × 10⁹/l (neutrophils 3.1, lymphocytes 2.1). He was commenced on ferrous sulphate 200 mg three times daily.
Two months later, he was still feeling lethargic and had developed numbness in his feet and difficulty concentrating. He returned to his general practitioner who found the following physical signs: pallor, angular cheilosis, splenic tip and soft sensory signs in both feet.
The haemoglobin was repeated and found to be 7.9 g/dl, MCV 114 fl, platelets 142 × 10⁹/l, WCC 3.6 × 10⁹/l (neutrophils 2.0, lymphocytes 1.6). Urea and electrolytes were normal. Serum calcium 2.4 mmol/l, phosphate 0.98 mmol/l, albumin 45 g/l, globulin 27 g/l, Alk Phos 110 U/l, ALT 39 U/l, AST 38 U/l and GGT 43 U/l. CXR was normal.
The patient was a divorced manual labourer who had lived on his own for about 10 years. He smoked 10 cigarettes a day and consumed 18 units of alcohol per week (never heavier than this). He had a mixed diet of meat and vegetables. In 1986 he had surgery for a bleeding peptic ulcer. He had had no more symptoms referable to this and had therefore not attended clinic since 1987. He was not on any regular medication.

(a) Give a differential diagnosis for the haematological findings.
(b) What are the possible pathophysiological bases for these findings and what investigations are indicated?
(c) What therapy would you recommend?

19. A 22-year-old woman attended antenatal clinic at 28 weeks' gestation in her first pregnancy. She felt tired and had had several nosebleeds and bruising recently. There had been no vaginal bleeding or abdominal pain. Fundal size was compatable with 28 weeks, and ultrasound confirmed the dates and revealed a normal pregnancy. She appeared pale but not icteric, there was no lymphadenopathy. Her BP was 110/70. A small haemorrhage was seen near the right optic disc.
Laboratory data at booking revealed a normal full blood count save for a marginally low platelet and neutrophil count. The patient was group O, Rhesus positive with no unexpected antibodies detected.
Repeat count at 28 weeks revealed Hb 8.4 g/dl, MCV 87 fl, WCC 2.5×10^9/l (neutrophils 0.7, lymphocytes 1.8), platelets 12×10^9/l. Blood film confirmed a true thrombocytopenia and neutropenia and revealed the presence of several promyelocytes; anisocytosis and schistocytes were also observed.
PT 19 s (control 15s), APPT 49 s (control 35 s), TT 20 s (control 11 s), fibrinogen 0.9 g/l.
Serum sodium 139 mmol/l, potassium 3.6 mmol/l, urea 8.4 mmol/l, creatinine 128 μmol, calcium 2.6 mmol/l, AST 36 U/l, Alk Phos 132 U/l. There was one plus of blood and protein on urine dipstick analysis.

(a) What is the most likely haematological diagnosis, and how can this be confirmed?
(b) What complication has developed, and how can this be confirmed?
(c) What management would you advise?

20. A 35-year-old man with haemophilia A was admitted for investigation of painless jaundice. He was a severe

haemophiliac and had received many different types of factor VIII over the years. He was seropositive for hepatitis B and C and HIV. He had not recently travelled abroad and had had no AIDS-defining illnesses. He had had no symptoms of cholecystitis.

On examination he was jaundiced with spider naevi. Splenomegaly 6 cm. Hepatomegaly 6 cm. No lymphadenopathy. Both knees were target joints and showed typical haemophilic arthropathy.

Haematology: Hb 12.9 g/dl, MCV 96 fl, platelets 53×10^9/l, WCC 10.7×10^9/l (neutrophils 8.4, lymphocytes 1.2) PT 27 s (control 14 s), APTT 52 s (control 35 s), TT 21 s (control 14 s), fibrinogen 1.2 g/l, D-dimers > 1000 ng/l.

Factor V 40%
Factor VII 35%
Factor VIII 1%
Factor IX 37%
Factor X 32%
Factor XI 41%
Factor XII 47%

Biochemistry: serum sodium 141 mmol/l, potassium 4.1 mmol/l, urea 4.2 mmol/l, creatinine 96 µmol/l, bilirubin 160 µmol/l, albumin 29 g/l, globulin 30 g/l, ALT 165 U/l, AST 272 U/l, Alk Phos 210 U/l.

Ultrasound of the liver was awaited.

(a) Summarize the haematological data and give a diagnosis.
(b) What is the cause for this?
(c) What advice would you give prior to invasive procedures?
(d) What treatment modality would improve hepatic pathology *and* the haemophilia?

CASE HISTORIES
ANSWERS

1. (a) 'Bence Jones only' myeloma, i.e. no serological evidence of a complete immunoglobulin paraprotein, but monoclonal light chains present in serum and urine.
   (b) Detection of Bence Jones light chains in urine. Repeat bone marrow aspirate with trephine.
   (c) 'Bence Jones only' myeloma is usually a more aggressive type of myeloma with a high incidence of renal and osteolytic damage.

The vast majority of myeloma patients possess a serological monoclonal paraprotein that is a complete immunoglobulin plus Bence Jones light chains. However, about 15% of myeloma patients have monoclonal light chains in serum and urine without a complete immunoglobin in the serum. Although Bence Jones protein (BJP) may be detectable by simple **dipstick** analysis, this is not always the case (Duffy, 1992). In the present case, urinalysis was positive for some time but this was difficult to interpret against a background of **hypertension**. However, myeloma develops over several years before it becomes clinically manifest and the earlier proteinuria may well reflect the presence of BJP. In the absence of biochemical evidence for renal damage it seems unlikely that the BJP excretion could account for the earlier hypertension. It is far more likely that the hypertension in this case reflects the higher incidence of this condition in Blacks. Although heterozygote Hb S can be associated with increased urinary infection and renal damage, this was a coincidental finding in this patient (up to 8% of native Africans are heterozygous for Hb S).

Myeloma frequently causes a **normochromic normocytic anaemia** with some degree of marrow failure which manifests as cytopenias. The marrow failure is probably a consequence of the myeloma damaging normal haemopoietic architecture and tissue. Note that folate deficiency and ring sideroblasts can also contribute to anaemia in myeloma.

The positive charge on paraproteins in myeloma can partially neutralize the negatively charged sialic acid residues on the erythrocyte surface. As a consequence, the electrostatic repulsion that keeps erythrocytes apart is diminished, leading to closer erythrocyte apposition and a more rapid ESR.

Osteoporosis alone may be found in 20% of myeloma patients. Although 60% of all patients have osteolytic lesions, about 80% of 'BJP only' patients have such lesions. However, myeloma is a very patchy disease and marrow aspirates frequently miss affected areas. It is important to perform a trephine biopsy in addition to an aspirate, to improve the diagnostic yield.

Much has been written about **prognostic factors** in myeloma. Durie and Salmon (1975) devised a system for assessing long-term outlook in these patients, based on the degree of anaemia, hypercalcaemia, uraemia, level of paraprotein in serum/urine and osteolytic damage. It is now felt that the single most important independent prognostic factor is the serum β_2-microglobulin level (Durie, 1988). This is part of the human leukocyte antigen (HLA) class I molecule and although concentrations increase during renal impairment, the degree of elevation of β_2-microglobulin remains an independent prognostic factor even in the presence of uraemia.

Duffy, T. P. (1992) 'The many pitfalls in the diagnosis of myeloma', *New England Journal of Medicine*, **326**: 394.

Durie, B. G. M. and Salmon, S. E. (1975) 'A clinical staging system for myeloma. Correlation of measured myeloma cell mass with presenting features, response to treatment and survival', *Cancer*, **36**: 842.

Durie B. G. M. (1988) 'Plasma cell disorders', *Recent Advances in Haematology*, **5**: 305–328.

Hoffbrand V. and Lewis, S. M. (1989) *Postgraduate Haematology*, 3rd edn, Oxford: Blackwell Scientific.

2. (a) Systemic lupus erythematosus (SLE), confirmed by antibodies to double-standard DNA.

(b) Lupus anticoagulant confirmed by anticardiolipin antibody titre and dilute Russell's viper venom test (DRVVT).
Haemolytic anaemia. Coombs' test has IgG specificity, probably warm type.
Mild neutropenia.
Postsplenectomy features in blood film plus mild lymphocytosis.

(c) Maintain thrombin time 4–5 times control value.

ITP has been recognized as an early herald for SLE for some years. However the thrombocytopenia of ITP is due to an autoantibody to the IIb/IIIa molecule on the platelet surface, whereas low platelet counts in SLE are usually due to immune complexes binding and causing destruction to the 'innocent bystander'.
Over 75% of patients with ITP respond to steroid therapy but relapse is not uncommon. If the patient has lost steroid responsiveness, then splenectomy is the preferred therapeutic modality in most cases – the majority of cases having a lasting response. Vaccination against *Pneumococcus* and *Haemophilus influenza* should be performed prior to splenectomy, and boosters given regularly thereafter.
The **lupus anticoagulant** occurs in about one-fifth of patients with SLE. The circulating antibody interferes with the tenase and prothrombinase clotting factor complexes binding to the platelet surface and prolongs the KCCT. At the same time, activation of protein C at endothelial thrombomodulin is disturbed by the antibody producing a prothrombotic tendency (Creagh and Greaves, 1991). The clinical antiphospholipid syndrome is recognized as an arterial or venous thrombosis (or recurrent miscarriage or thrombocytopenia) **plus** the presence of anticardiolipin antibody and/or a specific test for the functional effect of the anticoagulant, on more than two occasions (Harris, 1990). Detection of anticardiolipin antibody is now quite sensitive and specific. The prolonged KCCT seen with the lupus anticoagulant does not correct when normal plasma is mixed with the patient's plasma because the antibody binds to the elements of normal plasma as well. The DRVVT

activates factor X in the presence of small amounts of platelets, the presence of anticardiolipin antibody retards the clotting process. If massive amounts of platelets are added to the reaction mixture, the effect of the antibody is swamped ('platelet correction').

Pancytopenia is not infrequent in SLE and has an autoimmune basis. Haemolytic anaemia resulting from antibodies binding to the erythrocyte surface; thrombocytopenia and neutropenia resulting from immune complex mechanisms. Very rarely an aplastic type picture may be found. The effects of therapy should always be considered.

In this case, the blood film appearances are features of splenectomy; however, polychromasia and spherocytes suggest an ongoing haemolytic process. Warm autoantibodies are not uncommon in SLE and steroids are usually effective in improving the anaemia.

As the KCCT is already prolonged, **monitoring the effect of heparin** may be difficult. As the TT is only really influenced by fibrinogen or heparin, monitoring this parameter is to be preferred. The alternative of aiming to prolong the KCCT 1.5 to 2 times the patient's basal KCCT is second best in this situation.

Creagh, M. D. and Greaves M. (1991) 'Lupus anticoagulant', *Blood Reviews*, **5**: 162.

Harris, N. (1990) 'Antiphospholipid antibodies', *British Journal of Haematology*, **74**: 1.

3. (a) Mother is an α-thalassaemia heterozygote; fetus is an α-thalassaemia homozygote.

   (b) The Mother's DNA can be probed for deletions of the α-globin gene. Fetal blood sampling would reveal anaemia and the presence of Hb Barts (γ_4); DNA would reveal deletions in all α-globin genes.

   (c) To produce an α-thalassaemic homozygous fetus, the father must also be heterozygous for α-thalassaemia.

There are two functional α-globin genes on each chromosome 16. Deletions within a single gene occur in African races, whereas deletions within both genes on the same chromosome occurs more frequently in Chinese (and occasionally Mediterranean) races. Loss of one or two α-globin genes results in a microcytic and hypochromic blood picture, often with little effect on the Hb, although the red cell count is usually elevated. Hb electrophoresis reveals no abnormality because Hb A_2 and Hb F are produced in normal amounts. Loss of 3 α-globin genes produces a hypochromic microcytic anaemia with splenomegaly; Hb electrophoresis demonstrates Hb A, A_2, H ($β_4$) and some Barts ($γ_4$), the latter two resulting from impaired α-chain synthesis. When all 4 α-genes are deleted, only $γ_4$ can be produced in the fetus and this results in profound ineffective erythropoiesis and cardiac failure (hydrops fetalis), often leading to death in utero. The presence of a hydropic fetus is usually associated with pre-eclampsia.

The diagnosis of α-thalassaemia should always be considered when microcytic indices are present without iron deficiency. If Hb electrophoresis reveals a normal Hb A_2 (i.e. not β-thalassaemia), the diagnosis of α-thalassaemia is almost certain (although βδ-thalassaemia is a less likely possibility). Examination of globin chain synthesis reveals reduced α-chain production; this technique is labour intensive and has been superseded by genetic analysis of the α-globin genes.

The importance of α-thalassaemia is mainly in terms of preventative medicine. The identification of individuals with microcytic indices who are not iron deficient enables informed genetic counselling. The diagnosis of either α- or β-thalassaemia carriers is nowhere more important than in pregnancy, a situation in which rapid and accurate diagnosis is vital.

The possibility of anti-RhD causing hydrops in this case is excluded by the phenotype of the mother who is Rh D positive, and therefore cannot make anti-RhD. RhD negativity is 15% in the UK but only 0.2% in China.

Hoffbrand, V. and Lewis, S. M. (1989). *Postgraduate Haematology*, 3rd edn, Oxford: Blackwell Scientific.
Weatherall, D. J. and Clegg, J. B. (1989). *The Thalassaemic Syndromes*, Oxford: Blackwell.

4. (a) Hodgkin's lymphoma. Lymph-node biopsy.

(b) AIDS – HIV serology.
Tuberculosis – sputum examination, Mantoux test.

N.B. Bronchoscopy may be helpful in each of these situations but will not necessarily yield a definitive diagnosis.

Although many patients with Hodgkin's disease (HD) present with isolated lymphadenopathy and are curable, some patients present with very aggressive disease (Urba and Longo, 1992). Such cases are usually lymphocyte depleted or aggressive nodular sclerosing in histological type, with Stage IV disease. Involvement of lung, liver, gut, CNS and bone are all documented, although only 5% of cases at presentation have a positive marrow trephine. Treatment of **pulmonary disease** is often problematic, as it may not be clear whether the CXR changes are due to lymphoma plus or minus infection. CT scanning is not always that helpful, but bronchoscopy may provide microbiological and histological help. The presence of B symptoms (fever, weight loss, night sweats) will often give a clue to the lymphomatous nature of the illness, and response to chemotherapy (symptoms and radiology) is suggestive that lymphoma is the predominant element. This type of patient may make a good response to initial chemotherapy regimens, although the likelihood of relapse makes him a candidate for autologous marrow transplantation following remission. Harvesting peripheral blood stem cells and the use of growth factors has resulted in newer, transplantation strategies, which are under evaluation (Linch, 1988). Several groups have attempted to produce prognostic scores in HD, common factors are stage, histology, age, chest disease, ESR, serum albumin, Hb and lymphocyte count.
In this case, the clues to HD rather than the other diagnoses are the haemolysis, thrombocytosis and eosinophilia. NHL may cause haemolysis, but marrow involvement is usual, and eosinophilia and thrombocytosis are rare. Further more, pulmonary involvement with NHL is less common

than in HD (Filly *et al.*, 1976). The patient has no apparent HIV risk factors. Pulmonary TB is a possibility now that the incidence is increasing, but the non-tender nature of the lymphadenopathy and the haematological features point away from this diagnosis.

Filly, R., Bland, N. and Costello, R. A. (1976) 'Radiographic distribution of intrathoracic disease in previously untreated patients with Hodgkin's disease and non-Hodgkin's disease', *Radiology*, **120**: 277.

Linch, D. C. (1988) 'The management of Hodgkin's disease and non-Hodgkin's lymphoma', *Recent Advances in Haematology*, **5**: 211–242.

Urba, W. J. and Longo, D. L. (1992) 'Medical progress: Hodgkin's disease', *New England Journal of Medicine*, **326**: 678.

5. (a) History of drug ingestion, viral illness, solvent/benzene exposure, family history of haemic disease, radiation.
   (b) Hypoplastic presentation of AML.
   (c) Serum sickness – arthralgia, pulmonary infiltrates, glomerular damage, rashes. Steroids are given prophylactically to reduce these toxicities.

Acute leukaemias may present with a hypoplastic marrow. This is more common in childhood ALL, but also occurs in adult AML and ALL. Aplastic anaemia itself may also demonstrate clonal evolution to acute leukaemia (via PNH or MDS). There were no features of PNH or MDS in this case and she was a *de novo* hypoplastic presentation. The leukaemic deposits may not be readily evident in the biopsy, but blasts should aways be specifically sought in hypoplastic trephines. The administration of G-CSF resulted in the myeloid clone expanding in to the circulation as myeloblasts; repeat marrow aspirate showed this.
Antilymphocyte globulin (ALG) is raised in rabbits or horses by injecting human lymphocytes. The resultant serum is highly allergenic and produces severe toxicities, which can be ameliorated with prophylactic steroids. ALG (± cyclosporin A) is standard treatment for aplastic anaemia; it may take a few months to become effective. ALG can work sufficiently well to defer allogeneic transplantation; however, the majority of these patients require BMT or end up with severe marrow failure and then can only be treated with supportive measures alone.

6. (a) Thrombotic thrombocytopenic purpura (TTP).
   (b) Thrombocytopenia associated with
       (i)   marrow infiltration, e.g. leukaemia, myeloma
       (ii)   infection
       (iii) ITP.
   (c) Bone marrow to exclude infiltration. Plasmapharesis
       plus replacement with FFP.

TTP is a syndrome featuring fever, thrombocytopenia,
microangiopathic haemolytic anaemia, neurological
phenomena and mild renal impairment – the clotting screen
is only mildly, if at all, deranged. The syndrome has been
associated with pregnancy, the oral contraceptive pill,
cyclosporin A, mitomycin and urinary infections. It may
have a sudden or insidious onset.
The pathology results from microthrombi within the
capillary bed but it is unclear whether this arises from
endothelial wall damage or increased platelet aggregation.
Plasma analysis suggests that the syndrome results from
reduced endothelial prostacyclin production; other workers
suggest that a platelet-agglutinating factor associated with
very large von Willebrand's multimers causes platelet
clumping. Such capillary damage in different tissues results
in the variety of clinical features observed.
The syndrome is very variable in its manifestations.
Neurological complications include fits, focal episodes,
coma and psychosis, all of which may be fluctuating in
nature. Microangiopathic haemolysis results from damage
to erythrocytes as they pass through microthrombotic
meshes within capillaries. Renal damage is usually mild and
proteinuria is common.
Although the present case is hypertensive and therefore
predisposed to developing transient ischaemia attacks, the
thrombocytopenia requires explanation; thrombocytopenia
is rarely associated with methyldopa. The clues are in the
previous history of a urinary tract infection and the
presence of schistocytes on the blood film.
The administration of FFP generally improves symptoms
whilst **plasmapheresis** is being organised. As this syndrome
has a definite mortality, plasmapheresis should be

performed early with a view to getting rid of potential causative molecules. Some patients respond well to such therapy and some make a gradual improvement; however, others succumb rapidly.

Hoffbrand, A. V. and Lewis, S. M. (1989) *Postgraduate Haematology*, 3rd edn, Oxford: Blackwell Scientific.

7. (a) Blood film examination to exclude platelet clumping and to check erythrocyte morphology. Clotting studies (PT, APPT, fibrinogen). Bone marrow aspirate. Platelet associated immunoglobulin (Pl IgG). Antinuclear factor and lupus anticoagulant. Quantitation of proteinuria. Fasting blood glucose.
   (b) ITP. (?Glucose intolerance.)
   (c) ITP, 'gestational thrombocytopenia', pre-eclampsia, hemolysis, elevated liver enzymes, low platelets (HELLP) syndrome, disseminated intravascular coagulation, thrombotic thrombocytopenic purpura/haemolytic uraemic syndrome, SLE, antiphospholipid syndrome, drug ingestion, HIV, type IIb von Willebrand's disease (vWD) marrow infiltration (e.g. leukaemia, lymphoma, cancer), other causes of thrombocytopenia seen in non-pregnant situations.
   (d) Confirm the diagnosis as far as possible. Once ITP is confirmed, prednisolone, 1 mg/kg orally, should be commenced if there is evidence of bleeding or platelets are unacceptably low.

DIAGNOSIS. ITP is the commonest cause of thrombocytopenia in the first and second trimester, and pregnancy often worsens the condition. Getting the diagnosis right is important because specific therapy is required. Ninety per cent of ITP patients have Pl IgG, this crosses the placenta and can result in potentially fatal fetal/neonatal thrombocytopenia requiring antenatal intervention. Unfortunately, neither maternal Pl IgG levels nor maternal platelet counts are reliable predictors of the neonatal count. The diagnosis of ITP is very likely if high levels of Pl IgG are found with platelet counts $< 50 \times 10^9/l$ and a bone marrow demonstrating plentiful megakaryocytes with no evidence of marrow malignancy; however, other potential causes must be actively sought. Pl IgG is not specific for ITP; thrombocytopenias associated with infections and inflammatory disorders may also demonstrate antibodies.

The term 'gestational thrombocytopenia' refers to mild/moderate thrombocytopenia in an otherwise healthy pregnancy with no prior history of ITP (McCrae *et al.*, 1992). Although Pl IgG may be detectable, the risk of neonatal thrombocytopenia is not increased and antenatal intervention is deemed inappropriate. The single most important factor in making this diagnosis is excluding antecedent ITP by questioning about previous bleeding tendency and the course of previous pregnancies. Although there was no previous history of ITP in the present case, a count of 36 makes gestational thrombocytopenia unlikely.

Thrombocytopenia can be an early feature of **pre-eclampsia**. This results from accelerated platelet destruction due to increased platelet adherence to damaged endothelium and thrombin formation. Although the present case is a primigravida, she did not fit the definition of PET: her BP did not rise above 140/90, and proteinuria was mild (proteinuria > 0.3 g/day for PET). The **HELLP** syndrome is a variant of PET and includes: (a) microangiopathic haemolysis; (b) elevated liver enzymes and (c) thrombocytopenia < 100×10^9/l (Weinstein, 1982); this is usually in addition to mild to moderate PET. The present case had normal liver function and no microangiopathic change on the film, thus excluding HELLP.

The absence of systemic bruising/bleeding or uterine bleeding makes the diagnosis of **DIC** unlikely, although clotting studies are essential in this situation. Similarly, there are none of the classical features of **TTP/HUS** about this case (see elsewhere). Although vWF rises in pregnancy, vWD type IIb can be associated with worsening thrombocytopenia due to abnormal avidity of the vW molecule for platelets in this subtype of the disease. There are no features about this case which suggest SLE as an underlying diagnosis, although SLE often worsens in pregnancy and can be associated with thrombocytopenia.

The thrombocytopenia of HIV may appear in pregnancy (± Pl IgG) and needs to be considered if risk factors are present, e.g. multiple partners.

These potential causes of thrombocytopenia in pregnancy need to be excluded to ensure that the diagnosis of ITP is correct. However, marrow infiltration by leukaemia, etc., can present in pregnancy and marrow examination is mandatory, especially in more severe cases of thrombocytopenia. Clues to recent viral or parasitic infections or drug ingestion must also be sought.

MANAGEMENT. There is much discussion about the treatment of ITP in pregnancy and this stems from a reluctance to treat a woman who is otherwise well, and the uncertainty about risk to the fetus. If counts fall to 30×10^9 to 40×10^9/l or there is evidence of bleeding/purpura, then oral prednisolone should be commenced – two-thirds of patients respond. Intravenous immunoglobulin (IVIG) is an alternative and may be optimally timed a week prior to delivery. Splenectomy is quite hazardous but early in the second trimester seems safest time for surgery.

In ITP, it is impossible to predict the fetal platelet count from that of the mother; fetal blood sampling is therefore required. This may be performed by ultrasound-guided umbilical vein sampling, but may necessitate emergency caesarean section if complications arise. Other practitioners favour fetal scalp sampling once the head is engaged and the cervix dilated. This method can give rise to inaccuracies, but in experienced hands there is good correlation with umbilical vein sampling. Certainly, a normal fetal scalp platelet count in a thrombocytopenic mother is good evidence that the fetus is not thrombocytopenic. A fetal platelet count $< 50 \times 10^9$/l suggests that section is safest for the child; if it is $> 50 \times 10^9$/l, then vaginal delivery is probably safe.

Burrows R. F. and Kelton, S. G. (1993) 'Fetal thrombocytopenia and its relation to material thrombocytopenia', *New England Journal of Medicine*, 329: 1463–6.

McCrae, K. R., Samuels P. and Schreiber, A. D. (1992) 'Thrombocytopenia in pregnancy', *Blood*, 80: 2697–714.

Weinstein, L. (1982) 'Syndrome of haemolysis, elevated liver enzymes and low platelets; a severe consequence of hypertension in pregnancy',

American Journal of Obstetrics and Gynaecology, **142**: 159.
Winetrobe's Clinical Haematology, 9th edn (1993), London: Lea &
Febiger.

8. (a) Hepatic sequestration crisis.
   (b) Intravenous fluids, oxygen, analgesia (opiate),
       intravenous antibiotics, blood transfusion.
   (c) Difficulties in cross-matching the patient's serum
       against Caucasian blood.

Bony crises may presage the onset of sequestration crises
within the lungs, liver or pelvis. Such sequestration crises
are potentially fatal and need to be treated vigorously. In
children, splenic sequestration is a frequent cause of death
and parents are taught to search for splenic enlargement. As
the child grows, 'autosplenectomy' results in a small fibrotic
organ which is incapable of allowing sequestration. In adult
patients, the chest syndrome may follow rib infarction and
presents with increasing dyspnoea, pleurisy, hypoxia and
radiographic changes. The sequestration of blood within the
pulmonary vasculature results in further hypoxia and a
vicious circle is set up. This situation is extremely serious
and may be masked by opiate administration; management
with exchange transfusion or even extracorporeal
circulation may be necessary to halt the process. There are
no indications in the present case that sequestration is
occurring in the chest; however, hepatomegaly and elevated
liver enzymes give the clue to **hepatic sequestration**. Why
the process favours one organ as opposed to another is not
clear. Homozygous patients often have haemoglobins of
5–8 g/dl; a fall to 4.6 g/dl plus hypotension represents a
significant drop and reflects substantial sequestration within
the liver.
MANAGEMENT.   The standard regimens for treating
sickling crises are well known. Opiate addiction may result
in doctors being reluctant to give analgesia; however, the
patient should always be given the benefit of the doubt, as
this type of pain is very severe. Certain complications of
sickle disease require some form of blood transfusion,
especially if there is haemodynamic instability. Simple
top-up transfusion dilutes out the Hb S and may reduce

sickling; at the same time, total blood viscosity can be elevated and is potentially hazardous. The technique of exchange transfusion, exchanging normal blood for the patient's blood through a long-line, may be a superior way of reducing the amount of Hb S but is time-consuming and expensive. There are, however, certain well-defined indications for exchange transfusion, such as chest and girdle syndromes, priapism and cerebrovascular events. Sometimes this can be followed by a period of 'hypertransfusion' to maintain a lower Hb S level and reduce the risk of major complications recurring in subsequent months.

African blood is phenotypically different from Caucasian blood. *Plasmodium vivax* gains access to the erythrocyte via the Duffy antigen; loss of this red cell protein confers relative protection from the parasite. Thus, patients of African origin who receive blood products are liable to develop antibodies to antigens they do not possess. For this reason large amounts of blood are not always available for exchanging or hypertransfusion regimens and sometimes simple top-up has to be accepted. In a situation where there is difficulty obtaining blood for an emergency, the 'least incompatible' units on the cross match may sometimes be used under steroid cover.

Serjeant, G. R. (1993) 'The clinical features of sickle cell disease', *Clinical Haematology*, **6**: 93–116.

9. (a) Leukaemic transformation of Fanconi's anaemia.
   (b) Diepoxybutane (DEB) stress test.
   (c) Genetic counselling regarding this autosomally recessive disorder. The child's siblings should have a DEB stress test, and prenatal screening for this condition should be considered.

Fanconi's anaemia (FA) is associated with a number of somatic abnormalities: small stature, slow growth, microcephaly, abnormal thumbs, hyperpigmentation, depigmented spots, café au lait spots, strabismus, cryptorchism, mental retardation, deafness and horseshoe kidney (Schroder-Kurth *et al.*, 1989). These features can occur in a variety of permutations: such a variable phenotype reflects the chromosomal instability which is the fundamental abnormality in this disorder.

The blood count is normal at birth, but cytopenias develop at 5–10 years, or later. Thrombocytopenia and anaemia are more common than neutropenia. The marrow becomes increasingly hypoplastic. During this phase a myeloid leukaemic clone may become evident in the marrow ± blood; occasionally, as in the present case, AML may be the presenting feature. Any child presenting with AML should be considered as a possible case of FA. There is also an increased risk of non-haemic malignancies in affected individuals.

The chromosomal instability may be due to a number of factors, e.g. a reduction in DNA ligase activity or a reduction in superoxide dismutase activity allowing superoxide damage to DNA (Gordon-Smith and Rutherford, 1989). This results in spontaneous chromosomal damage and increased sensitivity to certain agents. For example, incubation of the patient's cells with alkylators such as DEB *in vitro* results in marked chromosomal damage compared with healthy control cells. This forms the basis of the DEB stress test required in the diagnosis of the homozygous state and it is suitable for prenatal testing.

Median survival for all patients with FA is 25 years; however, survival in patients with an early onset and the highest DEB sensitivity is half this figure. The presence of other somatic abnormalities also affects prognosis.

MANAGEMENT.   Anabolic steroids will improve hypoplasia over several months in most cases of non-leukaemic FA. There are inevitable toxicities with this therapy and peliosis hepatis and hepatic carcinoma are well described. This therapy may 'buy time' in which to find a suitable donor for marrow transplantation. Patients presenting in a leukaemic phase require chemotherapy, and this is problematic against a background of hypoplasia and unstable chromosomes.

Bone marrow transplantation (BMT) is the best option for FA patients with early onset or aggressive disease. BMT is best performed using an HLA-identical sibling who does not have FA; alternatively, matched unrelated donors or non-HLA-matched family donors can be considered. It is not uncommon for parents to extend their families in an attempt to provide suitable donors.

Other inherited conditions associated with increased leukaemic risk include Down's syndrome, Bloom's syndrome and ataxia telangiectasia.

Gordon-Smith, E. C. and Rutherford T. R. (1989) 'Fanconi anaemia – constitutional, familial anaemia', *Clinics in Haematology*, 2: 139–152.

Schroder-Kurth, T. M., Auerbach, A. D. and Ode, G. (1989). *Fanconi Anaemia: Clinical, Cytogenetic and Experimental Aspects*, Heidelberg: Springer-Verlag.

10. (a) Absolute polycythaemia secondary to renal disease. The RCM had been reduced in to the normal range by the previous venesections and the plasma volume was reduced as a result of antihypertensive therapy. Pseudopolycythaemia was an incorrect interpretation of the data.

    (b) Renal ultrasound/imaging; renal biopsy.

    (c) Antithrombin III, protein C and protein S activity, antiphospholipid antibodies, lupus anticoagulant screen.

This case illustrates the danger of misinterpreting laboratory data in the face of an obvious cause for polycythaemia; such incorrect diagnostic labelling could result in serious therapeutic errors.

The initial history of DVT and hypertension may have suggested a prothrombotic disorder, but apparently a blood count was normal or not performed at that time.

Thrombotic problems can presage the onset of myeloproliferative disorders (Boughton, 1991) and have an increased incidence in hypertension and renal disorders. In this case, the hypertension may be associated with the renal disease rather than a feature of polycythaemia.

When he was admitted with his MI, this patient was certainly polycythaemic. In this situation (and others such as cerebrovascular events), reducing the haematocrit can be beneficial – this must be performed with the utmost caution because the provocation of hypotension can obviously worsen the situation. Once the patient is stabilized, venesection can be performed at the same time as infusing an equal volume of crystalloid to maintain isovolaemia. Venesection reduced the RCM, and in the present case brought it into the normal range. Interpretation of plasma volume also needs care, as this can be affected by dehydration, diuretic and antihypertensive therapy. Laboratory data should always be considered in the context of clinical data.

'**Pseudopolycythaemia**' (Gaisböck's or relative polycythaemia) is a syndrome affecting middle-aged overweight men who smoke and drink excessively and who are in stressful situations. The present case did not fit this classical picture. Further, it is perverse to make such a diagnosis in the face of renal pathology. It may be argued that true polycythaemia (primary or secondary) may cause renal damage with subsequent proteinuria, but this is not usually the case. It is worth noting that Gaisböck's polycythaemia can develop into true polycythaemia in up to 50% of cases, and may be associated with similar complications, for these reasons relative polycythaemia requires regular follow up and venesection may be necessary.

The RCM is expressed in terms of the red cell volume divided by body weight, i.e. ml/kg. Adipose tissue is poorly vascularized, thus obese individuals with a borderline high red cell volume have a large denominator for calculating the RCM, and this may then fall into the normal range. This situation is termed 'apparent polycythaemia' and is a potential source of error. Some authorities suggest that the RCM calculation should involve correction factors and be based on ideal body weight or lean body mass. This does not pertain to the present case as he has a good reason for being polycythaemic.

Any young person with a major thrombotic event deserves further prothrombotic work-up despite coexisting disease. Renal disease may allow protein C to be lost into the urine, and such a reduction to protein C level may account for the thrombotic tendency observed in patients with nephrotic syndrome.

The present case was shown to have mesangiocapillary glomerulonephritis and had a normal prothrombotic screen.

Boughton, B. J. (1991) 'Hepatic and portal vein thrombosis', *British Medical Journal*, **302**: 192–3.

11. (a) Hereditary spherocytosis (HS) with B19 parvovirus infection precipitating red cell aplasia.
    (b) Blood film, osmotic fragility, autohaemolysis, parvovirus serology.
    (c) HS – gallstones, leg ulcers.
        B19 parvovirus – polyarthralgia, fifth disease.

HS has a wide clinical spectrum and can present from the neonatal phase through to late in life. In children, jaundice and anaemia may be troublesome but often the child is 'more yellow than sick'. Alternatively, HS can present in adulthood, reflecting the fact that the individual has maintained a 'compensated' haemolytic state which has not produced symptomatic anaemia. Chronic excess bilirubin production usually results in cholelithiasis, often in early adulthood.
In normal individuals, **B19 parvovirus** infection may cause a transient drop of 1–2 g in the Hb. In patients with a compensated haemolytic state, such a stress cannot be tolerated and symptomatic anaemia may ensue with a slow recovery. The virus specifically infects erythroid progenitors via the P antigen, resulting in impaired proliferation. The myeloid series is relatively spared although mild neutropenia and thrombocytopenia may occur. In immunocompromised individuals, persistent infection may result in prolonged symptomatic anaemia.
DIAGNOSIS. In HS, spherocytes are present on the blood film but may only represent a few per cent. A raised MCHC should always give a clue to the diagnosis. During an aplastic phase, the film may not be truly representative of HS. Osmotic fragility remains a routine method of making the diagnosis; preincubation of blood at room temperature for 24 hours before the test may make the test more sensitive. However, this test is neither very specific or sensitive – autoimmune haemolysis can give positive results.

The acidified glycerol lysis time, which measures the rate of haemolysis following the addition of acidified glycerol to the sample, has greater but not complete specificity for HS. Autohaemolysis is an alternative method.

In autohaemolysis, cells are incubated for 48 hours under sterile conditions at 37°C. Red cell membrane integrity depends on glucose metabolism within the erythrocyte. In HS the rate of glucose consumption is increased and autohaemolysis is higher than normal; when glucose is added to the incubation, autohaemolysis is near normal. In inherited anaemias due to glycolytic enzyme deficiency, abnormal autohaemolysis is not normalized by additional glucose as the glucose cannot be utilized due to a metabolic block. This can provide useful information in terms of further lines of investigation.

The pathology of HS lies within the instability of the red cell membrane, which results from reduced rather than dysfunctional α-spectrin production. This results in a decreased surface area being occupied by the cytoskeleton, which destabilizes the lipid bilayer. Part of the membrane is lost and the cell takes on a spherocytic shape. Cell deformability is reduced and entrapment within the splenic circulation results in further cell damage. For this reason, splenectomy may increase the Hb in HS, although the number of spherocytes on the film increases.

Hoffbrand, A. V. and Lewis, S. M. (1989) *Postgraduate Haematology*, 3rd edn, Oxford: Blackwell Scientific.

Palek, J. (1987) 'Hereditary elliptocytosis, spherocytosis and related disorders', *Blood Reviews*, 1: 147–68.

12. (a) CLL with associated folate deficiency (related to pemphigus?) and a monoclonal band.
    (b) Paraneoplastic pemphigus associated with CLL.
    (c) Biopsy of skin lesions with immunofluorescence studies.

There are certain features of this rash which point towards **pemphigus**: mouth lesions and a positive Nikolski's sign. About 90% of patients with pemphigus will develop lesions of the mucous membranes, whereas pemphigoid rarely affects these parts. Although some lesions in this patient were tense, the majority were flaccid with a positive Nikolski's sign, suggesting pemphigus.

Pemphigus occurs more commonly in people of Mediterranean extraction and may follow drug ingestion (e.g. penicillin, penicillamine, captopril). On biopsy, the lesions occur in a suprabasilar position with acantholysis. Immunoflourescence reveals IgG in the stratified squamous epithelium. It is thought that local release of plasmin produces proteolytic cleavage of cell to cell junctions resulting in acantholysis.

The association of pemphigus with neoplasia is established in both lymphoid and non-lymphoid malignancies (Anhalt *et al.*, 1990; Younus and Ahmed, 1990). The skin lesions may present before or after the malignancy becomes evident.

Stevens–Johnson syndrome is unlikely in the present case as the patient was not febrile and was relatively 'well'; target lesions were also few in number.

Folate deficiency can occur in most haematological malignancies and haemolytic states. The additional stress of pemphigus in this case of CLL has compounded the drain on folate stores – this has lead to a macrocytic anaemia. Although Coombs'-positive haemolysis may raise the MCV slightly if reticulocytes are plentiful, polychromasia was not a feature in the blood film of this patient. Marrow failure consequent to advancing disease or in relation to treatment may result in anaemia, but thrombocytopenia/neutropenia would also be expected. The patient has also developed an IgG monoclone; this occurs in up to 10% of CLL patients. There is a degree of suppression of the normal immunoglobulins by the cells producing this monoclonal IgG, and this may contribute to dysregulation of the immune system, resulting in increased risk of infection, neoplasia and autoimmune phenomena.

Anhalt, G. J. , Kim, S. C., *et al.* (1990) 'Paraneoplastic pemphigus – an autoimmune mucocutaneous disease associated with neoplasia', *New England Journal of Medicine*, **323**: 1729–35.

Younis, J. and Ahmed, A. R. (1990) 'The relationship of pemphigus to neoplasia', *Journal of the American Academy of Dermatology*, **23**: 498–502.

13. (a) Gaucher's disease with hypersplenism.
    (b) Bone marrow examination for Gaucher cells;
        leucocyte β-glucosidase level.

Gaucher's disease is an autosomal recessive disease found most commonly in people of Jewish extraction. It is caused by a deficiency of the enzyme glucocerebrosidase (glucosylceramidase, β-glucosidase), an enzyme involved in lipid degradation. Deficiency of this enzyme results in an accumulation of insoluble glucocerebroside within macrophages. There are a number of mutations described within the gene, most resulting in a change at amino acid 370 within the enzyme. The heterozygous state may confer a relative resistance to tuberculosis.

There are three common **clinical phenotypes**. Type I, which accounts for > 90% of cases, is often relatively asymptomatic and may present with mild splenomegaly ± hypersplenism in middle life. Hepatic fibrosis may occur. Neurological signs are not a feature. Bone infarcts or fractures may occur and aseptic necrosis of the femoral head has been described. This is compatible with a normal life-span. Type II presents with fulminant neurological damage with spasticity, strabismus and retroflexion of the head; death occurs within the first year or so. Type III presents in later childhood with more progressive neurological damage and a longer course. The case described corresponds to a type I phenotype. He has married a homozygous or heterozygous woman and produced a severely affected child (type II phenotype); the change in severity is probably accounted for by a mixture of genetic mutation types. Similarly, the type III phenotype of the cousin probably corresponds to yet a different mixture of mutations.

The hepatomegaly and raised liver enzymes in the present case is probably associated with a degree of liver damage; liver biopsy would reveal Kupffer cells full of glucocerebroside. The mild pancytopenia and splenomegaly point towards a bone marrow aspirate in the first instance. In fact, this showed a hyperplastic marrow with clumps of Gaucher's cells, which appear as large pale cells with an onion-layered appearance in the cytoplasm, and a small eccentric nucleus. The definitive diagnosis requires the measurement of a leucocyte β-glucosidase level.

The vast majority of patients are asymptomatic and require no treatment. Splenectomy (partial or full) may improve hypersplenism or discomfort but may accelerate the disease at other sites. Bone marrow transplantation has been less commonly performed since the advent of enzyme therapy. The commercially available form of glucocerebrosidase is slightly modified to improve its efficiency, and is given to patients with the non-neurological form of the disease. The enzyme is purified from human placenta, and is given as a fortnightly intravenous injection (Cox, 1993). Great therapeutic benefit has accrued in many of these patients.

Beutler, E. (1991) 'Gaucher's disease', *New England Journal of Medicine*, **325**: 1354–60.

Cos, T. M. (1993) 'Gaucher's disease: a brand leader', *The Lancet*, **342**: 694–5.

14. (a) Non-Hodgkin's lymphoma (NHL) with obstruction of both ureters/renal infiltration by NHL. Coombs'-positive haemolytic anaemia.

(b) Lymph node biopsy and CT scan of chest and abdomen with particular importance attached to the lower urinary tract.

NHL can produce several abnormalities in immune function, this is a consequence of dysregulation of normal B cell activity. Autoantibodies to red cells or other proteins may be a presenting feature. Polyclonal rises in immunoglobulin fractions and cryoglobulins may also be a feature. There is no monoclonal band and no mention of Bence Jones protein (BJP), so this makes myeloma very unlikely; furthermore, immune haemolysis in myeloma is extremely rare. The reticulocytosis produces polychromasia on the blood film and is a response to the haemolytic process; similarly the erythroid hyperplasia is a feature of active haemolysis.

Tuberculosis is a possibility here but the generalized
lymphadenopathy and lack of pulmonary disease make
this unlikely in this situation. The cough and mild
dysphagia can be attributed to the superior mediastinal
node mass, although there are no other features of
superior vena caval obstruction.
NHL may cause renal damage by several mechanisms.
Nodal compression of pelvic structures such as the
ureters can be a presenting feature of NHL; dilation of
the calyces in this case makes this likely and imaging at
the lower end of the urogenital tract will confirm this.
Interstitial infiltration of the kidneys by lymphoma
causes 'large kidneys' on ultrasound but not usually
obstruction. Other causes of renal damage in NHL
include sepsis, hypercalcaemia, tumour lysis and drugs.

15.(a) Glucose-6-phosphate dehydrogenase (G6PD)
deficiency with intravascular haemolysis due to
malaria and primaquine; renal failure has developed
due to sustained haemoglobinuria.
(b) G6PD assay on reticulocyte-depleted blood.
(c) Stop primaquine but continue quinine. Assess renal
status and attempt a forced diuresis if possible.

G6PD deficiency occurs in Africa, Asia, the Arabian
peninsula and the Mediterranean. It may cause very little
in the way of symptoms unless an oxidizing stress
decompensates erythropoiesis. This patient has
obviously had very little in the way of significant
oxidizing stresses as he has not had any major haemolytic
crises previously.
Severe infection is a potent cause of haemolysis in
G6PD-deficient individuals. Intravascular haemolysis
results in haemoglobinuria rather than haematuria. This
was mistakenly attributed to the malaria itself; however,
it is only *falciparum* that produces haemoglobinuria in
the presence of normal amounts of G6PD enzyme. The
oxidizing stress was compounded by the addition of
primaquine as therapy (chloroquine and quinine are
relatively safe agents). The renal failure is a consequence
of prolonged haemoglobinuria.

Young **reticulocytes** have a higher level of G6PD than older erythrocytes; if they are included in the enzyme assay, they can artificially elevate the level of G6PD. Consequently, blood is depleted of reticulocytes before the assay. The enzyme is assayed by reacting cells in a spectrophotometer in the presence of a specific substrate. Therapy consists of treating the infection but removing primaquine as a potential agent. Although primaquine can be used at lower doses in G6PD deficiency, it is probably best to substitute a different antimalarial in the face of renal failure. Careful hydration and assessment of central venous pressure/renal status is required to optimize renal function.

There are many different gene point mutations resulting in G6PD deficiency. The commonest African form (A –) produces a relatively mild phenotype, Mediterranean forms are often more severely affected. Heterozygotes rarely have significant problems. Once identified patients should be counselled about medication and implications for their family.

Hoffbrand, A. V. and Lewis, S. M. (1989) *Postgraduate Haematology*, 3rd edn, Oxford: Blackwell Scientific.

16. (a) Hepatic vein thrombosis, Budd–Chiari syndrome. Hepatic venography.
    (b) Paroxysmal nocturnal haemoglobinuria (PNH). The Ham's test or an acidified sucrose lysis test would confirm PNH. The absence of DAF and C8 binding protein can be demonstrated on erythrocytes.
    (c) Full but careful anticoagulation with monitoring for hepatic failure.

The cellular abnormality in PNH is loss of phosphatidyl inositol-linked structures at the cell membrane. In particular, DAF, C8-binding protein, FMLP receptor and immunoglobulin receptor are lost. The consequence of this is that complement accumulates on cell membranes and is not broken down. This can lead to erythrocyte membrane damage and platelet hypersensitivity to thrombin, resulting in platelet aggregation.

Hepatic vein thrombosis can be a presenting feature of PNH, frequently with non-specific abdominal pains. The classical features of hepatomegaly, jaundice and ascites are typical in this case, as is the sparing of the caudate lobe (which has a separate venous drainage). There are no clues to an infective or hepatic cause for these features. Presentation of the Budd–Chiari syndrome may be fulminant or of a more insidious nature; in the present case, a gradual, more moderate thrombotic process is more likely to have been occurring over some months. Anticoagulation with heparin is indicated to prevent further thrombosis, but heparin has been reported to promote further platelet aggregation in some individuals. Conversion to warfarin will need to be cautious in view of the prolonged PT. In fulminant Budd–Chiari syndrome thrombolytic therapy maybe life-saving. Careful monitoring of the patient for hepatic failure will be necessary – hepatic transplantation is hazardous under these circumstances.

Thromboses can occur in other sites such as brain (note the patient's headaches), kidneys, splanchnic bed, skin and peripheral veins (note the DVT). This thrombotic tendency results from increased platelet aggregation, and maybe the release of thrombophilic substances from disrupted erythrocytes.

PNH may present with pancytopenia/marrow hypoplasia or haemolysis (or a mixture of both). In the present case, the marrow trephine is hypoplastic and this accounts for the pancytopenia. There is no evidence of haemolysis as the blood film is not polychromatic. In classical PNH, there are no typical abnormalities in the clotting profile. PNH is a clonal disorder and may evolve as a response to hypoplasia/aplasia, it can also be associated with the development of acute leukaemia. In other patients, haemolysis is the predominant feature; this may be chronic or be precipitated by acute infections. Only a small number of patients actually describe red urine on waking (this is a sleep-dependent rather than diurnal process). The phenomenon of nocturnal haemoglobinuria may be explained by small

falls in the blood pH or increased endotoxin absorption
from the gut resulting in increased activation of
complement, resulting in erythrocyte fragility.
The basis of the **Ham's test** is acidification of the serum
resulting in complement activation and lysis of PNH but
not normal erythrocytes. Sucrose lysis time is less
sensitive and results from hypotonic sucrose solution
activating complement.
The treatment of PNH is mainly supportive. For patients
with hypoplasia/aplasia bone marrow transplantation is
an option. For patients with prolonged haemolysis, iron
deficiency may result from prolonged haemoglobinuria
and haemosiderinuria, this may compound anaemia.
Blood transfusion should be with plasma-reduced blood
or washed red cells to reduce infusion of donor plasma
complement.

Wintrobe's Clinical Haematology, 9th edn (1993), London: Lea &
 Febiger.
Rosse, W. F. (1989) 'Paroxysmal nocturnal haemoglobinuria: the
 biochemical defects and the clinical syndrome', *Blood Reviews*, **3**:
 192–201.

17. (a) T gamma-lymphocytosis (large granular lymphocytosis)
       with neutropenia and seropositive rheumatoid disease.
       Felty's syndrome is unlikely. Amyloid.
   (b) Bone marrow aspirate to estimate marrow content of
       lymphocytes. Phenotyping lymphocytes with
       monoclonal antibodies. Analysis of blood and/or
       marrow lymphocyte population for T cell receptor
       gene rearrangement.
   (c) No treatment in the first instance. Splenectomy is not
       indicated. If infections progress then oral
       chlorambucil may improve neutropenia.

Felty's syndrome occurs in severe longstanding
seropositive rheumatoid disease; nodules and extra-
articular manifestations are common. It is actually quite
rare, occurring in only 1% of patients with rheumatoid
disease, and the neutropenia usually follows many years
of disease. There is no lymphocytosis in the blood or
marrow. The cause of the neutropenia may be

antineutrophil antibodies or increased margination of neutrophils in the circulation. Although splenectomy can improve neutropenia, this is not always the case and recurrent infections may persist. More recently, G-CSF has been shown to be of benefit in some cases.

The present case does not fit the picture of Felty's syndrome because the clinical picture is not very severe or prolonged. The striking feature in the haematology, besides the neutropenia, is the lymphocytosis – the film revealed 'activated lymphocytes', which were actually large granular lymphocytes (LGLs). LGLs can form about 10% of lymphocytes in healthy individuals, this goes up in viral episodes and inflammation. However, a persistent increase in LGLs suggests a lymphoproliferative process. LGLs may be either NK cells (CD2+,3–,8–,16+) or a subgroup of cytotoxic T cells (CD2+,3+,8+,16+) which do not possess NK function. LGL lymphoproliferations can have either phenotype, but only cells possessing CD3 (T cell receptor) can be analysed for T cell receptor gene rearrangement by restriction enzyme polymorphism techniques. The demonstration of a constant rearrangement rather than many rearrangements is the hallmark of a clonal T cell proliferation.

Patients with a T gamma-lymphocytosis of CD3+ LGLs may present as a form of seropositive rheumatoid arthritis; the clinical features are milder than those of classical rheumatoid disease. The arthritic history is usually not as long standing as in Felty's syndrome. Splenomegaly, antineutrophil antibodies and neutropenia are also common. Recurrent infections are a feature. LGLs are usually present in the blood but may be more obvious in the marrow, where maturation arrest of the myeloid series may also be found. It is apparent therefore that this syndrome could be confused with Felty's syndrome. However, splenectomy is of no use in this condition; chlorambucil or G-CSF are more appropriate. Chlorambucil can reduce the lymphocytosis and improve constitutional symptoms but has no effect on the arthritis itself. Progression of the disease to

lymphoma may well account for the association of
lymphoma and Felty's syndrome by physicians in a
previous era.

Campion, G., Maddison, P. J., Goulding, N. *et al.* (1990) 'The Felty
syndrome: a case-matched study of clinical manifestations and
outcome, serological features and immunogenetic associations',
Medicine, **69**: 69–80.
Loughran T. P. (1993) 'Clonal disease of large granular lymphocytes',
Blood, **82**: 1–11.
Snowden, N., Bhavnani, M., Swinson, D.R. *et al.* (1991) 'Large
granular T lymphocytes, neutropenia and polyarthropathy: an
underrecognised syndrome?' *Quarterly Journal of Medicine*, **285**:
65–76.

18. (a) Mixed iron and B_{12} deficiency; mixed iron and folate
    deficiency.
    (b) Post-gastrectomy iron and B_{12} deficiency resulting
    from loss of gastric production of acid and intrinsic
    factor – serum iron, ferritin, B_{12}, Schilling test (parts 1
    and 2). Blind-loop syndrome resulting in B_{12}
    deficiency with concomitant iron deficiency – ^{14}C
    breath test, serum iron, ferritin, B_{12}. Post-gastrectomy
    acquired enteropathy resulting in iron and folate
    malabsorption – serum iron, ferritin, red cell folate,
    jejunal biopsy.
    (c) Oral iron and/or folate replacement; intramuscular
    B_{12} therapy. Tetracyclines for blind-loop syndrome.

At presentation, this patient had a **mixed deficiency**
which resulted in a normal MCV – iron therapy
unmasked the associated folate/B_{12} deficiency; this
became evident as a sharp rise in the MCV. In such mixed
deficiencies, the marrow appears megaloblastic but iron
staining is reduced; in uncomplicated megaloblastosis
iron is plentiful in erythroblasts and stromal cell stores.
Iron absorption is optimal under acidic conditions and is
reduced following gastrectomy. Thus, many gastrectomy
patients are given iron replacement routinely. Similarly,
removal of large amounts of stomach will result in
reduced intrinsic factor secretion and reduced B_{12}
absorption – routine B_{12} replacement is often given
(quarterly) for life. This patient had had major gastric

surgery and was then lost to follow up, which resulted in him not having regular full blood counts. Serum iron, ferritin and B$_{12}$ will assist the diagnosis, but a part 1 Schilling test will demonstrate poor B$_{12}$ absorption. The part 2 Schilling test will be normal if B$_{12}$ deficiency is due entirely to removal of intrinsic factor-producing mucosa; however, the part 2 may not be normal if large amounts of blind-loop bacteria take up the oral dose of B$_{12}$ making it unavailable for binding to the administered intrinsic factor. Antibiotic therapy or reconstructive surgery may be the only way to improve B$_{12}$ absorption.

Following gastrectomy, malabsorption may result from damage to the jejunum consequent on exposure to gastric contents – iron and folate are affected primarily; B$_{12}$ may not be abnormal. In the present case, serum calcium, phosphate, protein and alkaline phosphatase were normal, suggesting that significant malabsorption is unlikely.

19. (a) Acute promyelocytic leukaemia (M3 subtype of AML). Bone marrow aspiration (this revealed replacement of normal marrow elements by many promyelocytes) and chromosomal analysis [this showed a (15;17) reciprocal translocation (typical of M3 subtype)].
    (b) Disseminated intravascular coagulation (DIC), confirmed by elevated D-dimers.
    (c) FFP to replace clotting factors, cryoprecipitate to increase fibrinogen and platelet infusion will all reduce the risk of further bleeding. The patient underwent elective section and the baby survived; the mother went on to receive AML chemotherapy successfully and received an allogeneic bone marrow transplant.

The M3 subtype of AML is associated with a slightly better survival than other types of AML; however, it is also associated with a high incidence of DIC, which may lead to a higher initial mortality. The DIC may be a consequence of promyelocyte enzyme release, resulting in damage to the clotting cascade; this process often worsens when chemotherapy is commenced, necessitating aggressive administration of blood products.

The blood film provides the clue in this case, as promyelocytes very rarely appear in the blood other than in M3 AML; even in leucoerythroblastic and CGL films, left shifting rarely goes beyond the myelocyte phase. Marrow failure results from proliferation of promyelocytes damaging normal haematopoietic elements, resulting in cytopenias. Recently, retinoic acid has been shown to differentiate leukaemic promyelocytes into neutrophils (which may remain part of the leukaemic clone) and reduce the risk of worsening DIC; standard chemotherapy can then be given more safely. Retinoic acid cannot be given in pregnancy because of its teratogenic effect. The use of retinoic acid is particularly interesting as the (15;17) translocation involves the retinoic acid receptor gene. Once remission is obtained and chemotherapy completed, some haematologists feel that transplantation should not be performed because the M3 subtype has a better survival than other types of AML.

The degree of **DIC** in M3 AML can be profound and patients with lower fibrinogen levels seem to do worse. Vigorous support is required to reduce bleeding. The present patient did not have excessive blood loss postoperatively but did require blood product support. Heparin may improve the DIC, but most practitioners do not use it.

Acute leukaemia in pregnancy provides a difficult management problem. In the first trimester there is a 30% chance of major fetal damage with chemotherapy, and termination of pregnancy may be selected. In the second and third trimesters this risk is much lower; however, where possible, it is probably wise to deliver the baby before commencing chemotherapy. There are, nevertheless, several reported cases of successful outcomes in pregnancy following chemotherapy.

20. (a) Reduction of all clotting factors with prolonged PT, APTT, TT and low fibrinogen. Thrombocytopenia. The diagnosis is DIC.
    (b) Advanced liver disease (chronic active hepatitis, cirrhosis or hepatoma).
    (c) Avoid such procedures if at all possible. If absolutely necessary, give vitamin K, FFP, cryoprecipitate, platelets and factor VIII.
    (d) Hepatic transplantation.

Reviewing the clotting data, DIC accounts for all the features. Liver disease alone, without DIC, could prolong the PT and APTT and dysfunctional fibrinogen could prolong the TT; thrombocytopenia and raised D-dimers suggest DIC. In vitamin K deficiency or obstructive jaundice, factors II, VII, IX and X would be reduced, with relatively normal amounts of V, XI and XII. Factor VIII is remarkably low due to the haemophilia itself.

Liver disease in haemophiliacs has long been recognized. Virtually all haemophiliacs who have had factor VIII that was not virally inactivated (1970s to mid 1980s) will be positive for hepatitis C (HCV); less than 5% are chronic carriers of hepatitis B surface antigen (HBsAg). Since viral inactivation procedures were introduced for factor concentrates, transmission of viruses has become an extreme rarity (donor selection has also contributed to this).

HCV is particularly important because it can cause chronic hepatitis in 45–81% of patients. The progression of the disease through chronic progressive hepatitis and chronic active hepatitis to cirrhosis has been debated, but there is little doubt that progression occurs, with a mean time to cirrhosis of 17 years. Hepatocellular carcinoma is 30 times more common than the background incidence. Although patients may be relatively asymptomatic initially, progressive liver failure adds to the mortality in haemophilia A, and cirrhosis is the primary or associated cause of death in 8–17% of haemophiliacs.

In early chronic hepatitis, IFN-α treatment can improve histology and transaminases substantially. Cessation of therapy results in evidence of inflamation returning. Liver transplantation is reserved for advanced rather than early liver disease. Reinfection with HCV occurs, and concomitant HIV will also complicate matters. However, a new liver produces enough factor VIII to cure the haemophilia.

DATA INTERPRETATION

DATA INTERPRETATION
QUESTIONS

1. A 34-year-old Caucasian woman attended antenatal clinic
   for booking in her first pregnancy. A splenic tip was felt,
   but no other abnormality. There was no family or drug
   history of note. She had had an episode of cholecystitis the
   previous year.
   Hb 8.9 g/dl, MCV 96 fl, MCH 32 pg, MCHC 36.5 g/dl,
   reticulocytes 10%, WCC 8.9 × 10⁹/l (neutrophils 4.5,
   lymphocytes 3.5), platelets 185 × 10⁹/l.
   Haemoglobin electrophoresis: normal.
   Serum iron, B$_{12}$ and folate: normal.
   Red cell antibodies and Coombs' test: negative.

   (a) What is the most likely diagnosis?
   (b) How would you confirm this?
   (c) What treatment is required during pregnancy?

2. A 23-year-old woman presented with abdominal pain
   which required laparotomy. The findings suggested small
   bowel ischaemia. Examination of the heart was normal and
   she was in sinus rhythm. There was no other family history
   or medical history of note. She was not on the oral
   contraceptive pill. Her FBC and clotting screen were
   normal. There was considerable difficulty heparinizing her
   postoperatively.
   She had had a left calf DVT whilst on the oral contraceptive
   at the age of 20.

   (a) What is the most likely diagnosis? Give an appropriate
       test.
   (b) Give a differential diagnosis and appropriate tests.

3. A 56-year-old man presented with a right calf DVT. He had previously been healthy and a non-smoker.
Hb 11.8 g/dl, MCV 89 fl, reticulocytes 6%, platelets 98 × 10⁹/l, WCC 3.4 × 10⁹/l (neutrophils 0.9, lymphocytes 2.1). Coombs' test: negative. Blood film showed polychromasia and anisocytosis.
Marrow aspirate showed active erythroid activity, normal amounts of megakaryocytes and reduced myeloid activity but no leukaemia or myeloma. Bone biopsy showed a normocellular marrow with no evidence of any malignancy.
PT 16 s (control 15 s), APTT 35 s (control 34 s).
CXR: normal.

(a) Suggest a diagnosis.
(b) Give 1 important test that is required.

4. A 45-year-old woman had a left DVT which was in need of heparinization. She had had 3 pregnancies and was slightly overweight. She had no other thrombotic risk factors. At diagnosis her FBC and clotting screen were normal. However, 6 days into intravenous heparin therapy (28,000 units/day) her platelet count fell to 15 × 10⁹/l, KCCT 50 s (control 27 s), PT 17 s (control 15 s), D-dimers normal, fibrinogen 2.6 g/l.

(a) What is the most likely diagnosis?
(b) How would you confirm this?
(c) What treatment would you recommend?

5. A 60-year-old woman with long-standing rheumatoid arthritis developed a large bruise over her left thigh. She was taking only NSAIDs.
FBC: Hb 10.6 g/dl, MCV 85 fl, platelets 195 × 10⁹/l, WCC 5.6 × 10⁹/l (neutrophils 2.9, lymphocytes 2.4). PT 13 s (control 14 s), KCCT 56 s (control 27 s), TT 13 s (control 11 s), fibrinogen 4.5 g/l. Platelet function tests revealed a typical aspirin defect.

(a) What is the most likely diagnosis?
(b) How could this be confirmed?

6. A 65-year-old woman was admitted with pneumonia. Hb 10.6 g/dl, MCV 109 fl, MCHC 37 g/dl, platelets 233 × 10⁹/l, WCC 13.5 × 10⁹/l (neutrophils 9.6, lymphocytes 3.4). Blood film: RBC agglutinates observed. Coombs' test: positive (complement but not IgG). Serum B₁₂ and folate: normal.

(a) What is the most likely diagnosis?
(b) How can this be confirmed?
(c) What advice would you give?

7. A 38-year-old woman presented to casualty with increasing drowsiness. A recent 2-week history of blurring of vision was obtained from her husband. She responded to pain but little else, and she had upper motor neurone signs on the left side of the body.
Hb 9.6 g/dl, MCV 85 fl, platelets 677 × 10⁹/l, WCC 255 × 10⁹/l (neutrophils 235, lymphocytes 2, metamyelocytes 6, myelocytes 8, promyelocytes 4). Plasma viscosity 1.57 mPa/sec (normal 1.5–1.7).
Serum sodium 142 mmol/l, potassium 3.7 mmol/l, urea 5.6 mmol/l, creatinine 102 μmol/l, calcium 2.46 mmol/l, bilirubin 16 μmol/l, ALT 26 U/l, GGT 17 U/l.

(a) What is the most likely diagnosis?
(b) What is the quickest way of confirming that diagnosis immediately?
(c) What therapeutic manoeuvre could be of benefit?

8. A 60-year-old woman complained to her general practitioner of lethargy. Her blood could revealed: Hb 7.6 g/dl, (MCV 95 fl), WCC 133 × 10⁹/l (neutrophils 3.5, lymphocytes 129), platelets 112 × 10⁹/l, reticulocytes 210 × 10⁹/l. Blood film revealed no evidence of acute leukaemia, but revealed polychromasia and smear cells.

(a) What is the most likely diagnosis and how can it be confirmed?
(b) Give 3 reasons why she may be anaemic, plus 3 revelant tests.

9. A 35-year-old haemophiliac had received AZT for 18

months. He had had one episode of PCP and an episode of candidal oesophagitis. He was taking AZT 200 mg q.d.s. [plus co-trimoxazole (Septrin) and fluconazole orally as prophylaxis].
FBC: Hb 11.8 g/dl, platelets 43 × 10⁹/l, WCC 2.1 × 10⁹/l (neutrophils 2.0, lymphocytes 0.7 – CD4 0.2, CD8 0.6).
Bone marrow aspirate: mild dysplastic features in all cell lines, megakaryocytes present in normal amounts.

(a) What is the most likely cause of his thrombocytopenia and how could this be verified?
(b) Give a differential diagnosis.

10. A 45-year-old woman had received a single unit of blood during her hysterectomy. Both patient and donor were group A, Rhesus-negative (*cde/cde* genotype). Cross-match had been compatible by enzyme and Coombs' techniques. A week later she noticed a yellow tinge in her eyes and felt feverish. Her general practitioner performed an FBC: Hb 10.4 g/dl, platelets 185 × 10⁹/l, WCC 9.1 × 10⁹/l (neutrophils 5.3, lymphocytes 2.8). Serum bilirubin 87 μmol/l, AST 31 U/l, ALT 20 U/l.
She had no significant previous history of note, and had had 3 normal pregnancies. She consumes on average 8 units of alcohol per week.

(a) What type of process has occurred?
(b) How can this be confirmed?

11. A 25-year-old Pakistani woman booked in at an antenatal clinic with her 3rd pregnancy. The previous 2 pregnancies (within the last 3 years) had been uneventful. She had a good diet of meat and vegetables, and did not smoke or drink. She lived with her husband and children, and had been resident in the UK for 10 years.
Hb 9.8 g/dl, RCC 5.5 × 10¹²/l, MCV 57 fl, MCH 19 pg, MCHC 29 g/dl, platelets 274 × 10⁹/l, WCC 9.3 × 10⁹/l (neutrophils 7.2, lymphocytes 2.0). ZPP 99 μmol/mol (normal range 20–80).

(a) What is the most likely explanation of these results?

(b) Give 2 further tests you would perform on the woman.

12. A 37-year-old man was admitted in an unconscious state. He responded to pain, full examination of the nervous system revealed no focal abnormalities. He had hepatomegaly (6 cm) and several spider naevi, but no splenomegaly. There were no signs of bleeding. Pulse 100/min (sinus rhythm); BP 140/85. He had crepitations at the right base.

Hb 14.6 g/dl, MCV 106 fl, WCC 4.5 × 10⁹/l (neutrophils 2.2, lymphocytes 2.1), platelets 10 × 10⁹/l. PT 19 s (control 15 s), APTT 38 s (control 36 s), fibrinogen 1.5 g/l. Serum sodium 141 mmol/l, potassium 4.1 mmol/l, urea 3.5 mmol, creatinine 103 μmol/l, bilirubin 45 μmol/l, AST 230 U/l, GGT 312 U/l.

Information from his general practitioner revealed that he had a history of alcohol abuse, was on no medication, lived by himself and worked as a taxi driver.

(a) What is the most likely diagnosis?

(b) What immediate test would be useful?

(c) What other haematological investigation may be of help?

13. A 58-year-old man had had a panproctocolectomy for carcinoma (Duke's stage C) with no macroscopic or scan evidence of hepatic metastasis. The operation had been relatively uneventful and he had received 3 units of stored whole blood. On the 10th postoperative day he had developed a temperature of 39°C and a generalized erythematous rash. He was commenced on intravenous cephalexin and metronidazole but the temperature persisted. Blood and wound cultures were all negative. CXR and abdominal ultrasound revealed no evidence of infection or subphrenic collection. Colostomy produced persistent diarrhoea.

On day 14 his liver function had deteriorated – bilirubin 172 μmol/l, AST 463 U/l, ALT 385 U/l, Alk Phos 482 U/l. Liver ultrasound showed no evidence of abscess, and cholangiogram revealed no evidence of ascending cholangitis. Although his haematology was normal preoperatively, pancytopenia was now evident: Hb 10.5 g/dl, WCC 2.5 × 10⁹/l (neutrophils 0.4, lymphocytes 2.1), platelets 29 × 10⁹/l. Blood film confirmed cytopenias but showed no erythrocyte fragmentation. PT 26 s (control 15 s), APTT 40 s (control 38 s), fibrinogen 2.1 gm/l. Bone marrow biopsy revealed a hypocellular marrow, but all elements were observed – no leukaemia or malignancy was evident. Serology for hepatitis A, B and C, HIV and CMV were all negative. No antibodies were detected by transfusion screening.

He became hypotensive (unresponsive to pressor agents and blood products), developed acute respiratory distress syndrome (ARDS) and renal failure and died.

The patient was a journalist who had been previously well, on no medication. He was a non-smoker and drank 10 units of alcohol per week.

(a) What was the most likely diagnosis?
(b) How could this have been confirmed?

14. A 32-year-old man was diagnosed as having Stage IV Hodgkin's disease. His first course of chlorambucil/vincristine/procarbazine/prednisolone had been followed 1 week later by injections of adriamycin/bleomycin/vinblastine. There were no complications associated with this chemotherapy, and his cervical lymphadenopathy improved. During the next course of chemotherapy he had 2 grand mal seizures following the completion of his chlorambucil/vincristine/procarbazine/prednisolone (CLVPP). He made a complete neurological recovery from these fits but bilateral papilloedema was observed.

Hb 12.7 g/l, WCC 9.3 × 10⁹/l (neutrophils 7.2, lymphocytes 2.0), platelets 138 × 10⁹/l. Serum glucose 5.7 mmol/l, calcium 2.47 mmol/l, albumin 49 gm/l, sodium 139 mmol/l, potassium 4.2 mmol/l, urea 5.8 mmol/l, creatinine 128 μmol/l.

He works as a bus-driver and is on no medication. He gave a history of febrile seizures as a child.

    (a) What is the most likely diagnosis and how would this
        be confirmed?

    (b) What treatment would you recommend?

15. A 29-year-old woman in the 24th week of her first
    pregnancy had developed right sided pleurisy. On
    examination she had been found to have a pleural rub,
    normal heart sounds and no clinical evidence of a DVT.
    Hb 11.4 g/dl, WCC 10.5×10^9/l (neutrophils 8.3,
    lymphocytes 1.9), platelets 168×10^9/l. PT 16 s (control 16
    s), APTT 36 s (control 35 s). CXR revealed a right-sided
    plate atelectasis, and a V/Q scan confirmed a definite
    pulmonary embolus. She was commenced on intravenous
    heparin for 7 days, and warfarin was commenced on day 5
    of heparin therapy.
    She was discharged the day after her heparin finished, for
    follow up in the anticoagulant clinic. However, she was
    readmitted the next day with left-sided pleurisy and
    dyspnoea.

    (a) What do you think has happened and why?

    (b) How can this be avoided?

16. A 66-year-old retired policeman had had a leg ulcer for 2
    years; this had been attributed to venous stasis. The ulcer
    had been very slow to respond to standard measures. He
    presented to his doctor with worsening headaches. On
    examination he had a few cervical lymph nodes (2 cm
    diameter) and retinal vein engorgement.
    Hb 12.1 g/dl, WCC 9.2×10^9/l (neutrophils 3.1,
    lymphocytes 6.1), platelets 198×10^9/l. Blood film showed
    rouleaux and a few lymphoplasmacytoid cells. Serum
    sodium 138 mmol/l, potassium 3.7 mmol/l, urea 6.3 mmol/l,
    creatinine 112 µmol/l, calcium 2.54 mmol/l, albumin 39 g/l,
    globulin 42 g/l, ALT 35 U/l, AST 34 U/l, IgG 6 g/l, IgA
    2 g/l, IgM 30 g/l.

    (a) What is the most likely diagnosis and how would you
        confirm this?

    (b) What therapy would you recommend?

17. A 45-year-old woman presented with fatigue and difficulty coping with her job as a cleaner. On examination she was pale and slightly icteric; a splenic tip was felt but no lymphadenopathy.
Hb 5.7 g/l, WCC 6.4 × 10⁹/l (neutrophils 3.2, lymphocytes 3.0), platelets 48 × 10⁹/l. Blood film: polychromasia, occasional spherocytes and nucleated erythrocytes.
Coombs' test: positive (IgG).

   (a) What is the diagnosis?
   (b) What treatment is indicated?

18. A 25-year-old man had a compound fracture of his femur following a motor cycle accident. He had previously been healthy and on no medication. He required a pin-and-plate procedure and received 2 units of blood. His preoperative haematology showed: Hb 9.7 g/dl, WCC 13.2 × 10⁹/l (neutrophils 10.2, lymphocytes 2.9), platelets 634 × 10⁹/l. Blood film showed normochromic cells. His blood group was O, Rhesus positive (*CDe/CDe* genotype), and the 2 units of blood were cross-match compatible.
During his second unit of blood, he developed an anaphylactoid reaction with hypotension and bronchoconstriction, requiring adrenaline and hydrocortisone. The transfusion was stopped and blood samples examined. His Hb was 10.5 g/dl, WCC 13.9 × 10⁹/l (neutrophils 10.7, lymphocytes 2.6), platelets 648 × 10⁹/l. Coombs' test was negative. Re-examination of serum revealed no antibodies (other than anti-A and anti-B), and repeat cross-match was again negative. No HLA lymphocytotoxic antibodies were detected. Culture of the patient's blood and donor units were negative.

   (a) What is the most likely cause of the transfusion reaction?
   (b) What would you recommend regarding further transfusion?

19. A 64-year-old woman with myeloma had received seven courses of melphalan/cyclophosphamide and achieved plateau phase. Therapy was stopped and she remained well

for 8 months, when she was lost to follow up. Six months
after this, she was brought into casualty in a confused state.
She lived alone and did not smoke or drink alcohol. She was
on no medication.

On examination, she responded to deep pain. Pupillary
reflexes and fundi were normal. Other cranial nerves were
also normal. All reflexes were brisk and plantars were
extensor.

Hb 10.3 g/dl, MCV 92 fl, WCC 8.3 × 10⁹/l (neutrophils 6.5,
lymphocytes 1.8), platelets 148 × 10⁹/l. Serum sodium 143
mmol/l, potassium 4.6 mmol/l, urea 10.3 mmol/l, creatinine
237 μmol/l, glucose 5.3 mmol/l, calcium 2.56 mmol/l,
albumin 41 g/l, globulin 82 g/l, Alk Phos 145 U/l, ALT 26
U/l.

(a) What is the most likely diagnosis?
(b) What quick and simple test would support this
     diagnosis?
(c) Give a differential diagnosis.

20. A 64-year-old man was admitted to casualty with fever and
confusion. On examination he was pale and had a
temperature of 38.5°C. The tip of his right index finger was
gangrenous. He had 6 cm splenomegaly but no
hepatomegaly. There was no lymphadenopathy.

His wife gave a history of the patient pruning roses the week
before. The man had previously been healthy and was on no
medication. He was a non-smoker and was a retired banker.

Hb 8.2 g/dl, MCV 92 fl, WCC 2.5 × 10⁹/l (neutrophils 0.5,
lymphocytes 2.0, monocytes 0), platelets 63 × 10⁹/l. Blood
film showed a few 'activated lymphocytes'. PT 15 s (control
15 s), APTT 34 s (control 34 s). Bone marrow aspirate was
almost dry. A marrow trephine was performed and gently
rolled between two slides; this preparation was cellular with
all cell lines present, but there was no excess of blasts. The
trephine report was awaited.

(a) Suggest a diagnosis.
(b) What treatment would you recommend?

21. A 47-year-old man had been treated for late-onset asthma for 3 years with bronchodilators and inhaled steroids. Episodes had become more frequent and he had begun to produce a lot of sputum. He also gave a 6-month history of intermittent diarrhoea, abdominal distension and 1 stone weight loss. He had finger clubbing and bilateral basal crepitations. There was no lymphadenopathy or hepatosplenomegaly and no masses were felt in the abdomen.

Hb 10.6 g/dl, MCV 104 fl, WCC 9.1 × 10⁹/l (neutrophils 8.2, lymphocytes 0.8), platelets 297 × 10⁹/l. Blood film showed macrocytes and some acanthocytes. Serum urea and electrolytes: normal. Serum calcium 2.15 mmol/l, albumin 30 g/l, globulin 15 g/l, bilirubin 15 μmol/l, ALT 28 U/l, Alk Phos 214 U/l. HIV serology: negative. Sweat test: sodium 67 mmol/l, chloride 55 mmol/l (normal > 52 and > 40, respectively.

He was a married office worker with 2 children. He had never smoked and was a non-drinker.

(a) What is the most likely primary diagnosis and how would this be confirmed?
(b) Give 5 investigations for his abdominal symptoms.
(c) What treatment would you recommend?

22. A 65-year-old woman had been diagnosed as having pernicious anaemia at the age of 60 years (positive Schilling test which corrected with intrinsic factor; positive parietal and intrinsic factor antibodies). Since diagnosis she had received intramuscular B$_{12}$ quarterly. She had recently complained to her general practitioner of recurrent tiredness and sleepiness.

Hb 10.7 g/l, MCV 108 fl, WCC 7.3 × 10⁹/l (neutrophils 5.2, lymphocytes 2.0) platelets 198 × 10⁹/l. Reticulocytes 95 × 10⁹/l. Blood film showed macrocytosis but no polychromasia. Coombs' test: negative. Serum biochemistry: normal. Serum folate 4.1 μg/l, B$_{12}$ 982 μg/l, red cell folate 534 μg/l. Bone marrow showed macronormoblastic erythropoiesis but no evidence of megaloblastic change; myeloblasts were not increased; several ring sideroblasts were seen.

(a) What is the most likely cause of the anaemia?
(b) What diagnostic test should be performed?

23. A 21-year-old woman was seen in out-patients complaining of bruising and moderate menorrhagia for 6 months. Her general practitioner had prescribed iron tablets and she had taken no other medication. She was a housewife with 3 children. She had had no major illnesses.
Hb 11.4 g/dl, MCV 81 fl, WCC 7.3×10^9/l (neutrophils 5.2, lymphocytes 1.9), platelets 293×10^9/l. Blood film normal. PT 15 s (control 15 s), APTT 33 s (control 32 s), fibrinogen 3.7 g/l. Factor VIIIc 89%, vWF 87%, ristocetin cofactor 85%. Bleeding time 15 min (normal < 9 min). Bone marrow: normal.

(a) What is the most likely diagnosis?
(b) How can this be confirmed?
(c) What therapy should be considered prior to surgery?

24. A 5-year-old Asian boy had originally been referred to hospital for the investigation of 'pallor'. He had been growing normally and was symptom-free.
Hb 7.3 g/dl, RCC 5.4×10^{12}/l, MCV 65 fl, WCC 6.4×10^9/l (neutrophils 3.2, lymphocytes 2.4), platelets 284×10^9/l. Blood film showed microcytosis, target cells, poikilocytosis and anisocytosis. Haemoglobin electrophoresis: Hb F 98%, Hb A_2 2%.
Over the next few years he required an occasional transfusion and he developed splenomegaly (4 cm). He continued to grow normally with minimal symptomatology.
There was no significant family history of note.

(a) What is the most likely diagnosis?
(b) What consideration should be made regarding the origin of the disease in this individual?

25. A 54-year-old shopkeeper gave a 6-week history of dyspepsia related to food and fatty intolerance. Apart from a hernia repair he had been previously quite healthy. He lived with his family, drank alcohol once a week and

smoked 10 cigarettes per day. He was on no medication. On examination he had epigastric tenderness, but no hepatosplenomegaly. His chest and cardiac examination were clear.

Hb 12.4 g/l, RCC 6.6 × 10¹²/l, MCV 71 fl, WCC 27 × 10⁹/l (neutrophils 24.1, lymphocytes 2.6, monocytes 0.2), platelets 525 × 10⁹/l. Haemoglobin electrophoresis: Hb A 92.2%, Hb A₂ 2.7%, Hb F < 0.1%. Serum sodium 139 mmol/l, potassium 3.8 mmol/l, urea 8.4 mmol, creatinine 149 µmol/l, calcium 2.56 mmol/l, albumin 41 g/l, globulin 21 g/l, Alk Phos 115 U/l, ALT 28 U/l.

CXR: within normal limits.

(a) What is the most likely diagnosis and how can this be confirmed?

(b) What management would you recommend?

26. A 67-year-old man complained of tiredness and dyspnoea of effort. He had had a cholecystectomy at the age of 54 for gallstones. He was a retired sailor, smoked 20 cigarettes per day and drank 20 units of alcohol per week. He was on no medication.

Hb 8.6 g/dl, MCV 104 fl, WCC 4.5 × 10⁹/l (neutrophils 1.2, lymphocytes 3.2), platelets 56 × 10⁹/l. Blood film showed anisocytosis and hypogranular neutrophils. Serum urea and electrolytes were normal. Serum calcium 2.48 mmol/l, albumin 40 g/l, globulin 29 g/l, ALT 38 U/l, Alk Phos 117 U/l. A monoclonal IgGk of 19.3 g/l was demonstrated on immunoelectophoresis. The marrow aspirate was cellular and showed 18% myeloblasts with hypogranular myelopoiesis; megakaryocytes were present in normal numbers; erythroid activity was dysmorphic with 20% ring sideroblasts; there was no increase in plasma cells. The marrow trephine was in keeping with the aspirate and showed no increase in plasma cells.

(a) What is the diagnosis?

(b) What other marrow test may be of use?

(c) What management would you recommend?

27. A 56-year-old man had originally presented with a

macrocytic anaemia: Hb 7.8 g/dl, MCV 102 fl, platelets 138 × 10⁹/l, WCC 4.0 × 10⁹/l (neutrophils 2.1, lymphocytes 1.7). Vitamin assays were normal. Bone marrow had shown features of myelodysplastic syndrome without an excess of blasts, and cytogenetics had revealed a deletion of chromosome 5. The man had required blood transfusions intermittently over the next 3 years and received subcutaneous desferrioxamine to minimize iron overload. Three years after the initial diagnosis he presented with a rash over his face and upper trunk. The rash consisted of erythematous plaques with pustulation. He also developed episcleritis and intermittent pyrexia. Cultures of blood, urine and pustules were negative.
CXR: clear.
Hb 9.7 g/dl, MCV 97 fl, platelets 125 × 10⁹/l, WCC 4.2 × 10⁹/l (neutrophils 1.9, lymphocytes 2.3). Bone marrow biopsy showed myelodysplasia with no excess of blasts. Skin biopsy revealed neutrophil infiltration of the dermis but no vasculitis.

(a) What is the diagnosis?
(b) Suggest a treatment.

28. A 59-year-old woman was scheduled for a hemicolectomy for carcinoma of the colon. Hb 10.2 g/dl, MCV 76 fl, platelets 297 × 10⁹/l, WCC 10.7 × 10⁹/l (neutrophils 6.7, lymphocytes 3.2). Blood group O, RhD positive. During the operation she received 3 units of blood which had received a completely clear cross-match. She made a good postoperative recovery and was due to go home on day 10, when she noticed bruising over her legs and blood in the colostomy bag.
Hb 11.2 g/dl, MCV 80 fl, platelets 12 × 10⁹/l, WCC 13.2 × 10⁹/l (neutrophils 11.1, lymphocytes 2.3). PT 15 s (control 14 s), APTT 39 s (control 37 s), fibrinogen 3.7 g/l. Bone marrow was essentially normal with active megakaryocytopoiesis and no evidence of metastatic cancer. She had had 2 normal pregnancies. She had always been healthy, a non-smoker and was on no medication. She drank alcohol socially.

(a) What is the most likely diagnosis?
(b) What is the mechanism?
(c) What treatment would you recommend.

29. A 7-year-old boy was brought to his general practitioner because he had a swollen knee after playing football. His parents said that they had noticed that his knees and elbows tended to swell after moderate trauma. There was no recent history of infection or rash and he had not received any medication. There was no family history of note.
Hb 12.9 g/dl, MCV 89 fl, platelets 269 × 10⁹/l, WCC 8.7 × 10⁹/l (neutrophils 5.9, lymphocytes 2.1). PT 14 s (control 14 s), APTT 57 s (control 37 s), fibrinogen 3.2 g/l, factor VIIIc 89%, vWF 87%, RiCof 85%.

(a) What is the most likely diagnosis?
(b) What further tests would you perform?

30. A 57-year-old woman had been attending out-patients with primary proliferative polycythaemia (PPP) for 4 years. She had received venesections and latterly hydroxyurea. The latter agent was controlling her haemoglobin but her WCC and platelets were progressively rising. Blood film showed left-shifted myeloid series, occasional nucleated red cells and poikilocytes. Her spleen had increased from 4 to 10 cm. A bone marrow aspirate was dry.

(a) Name the 2 most likely causes of these developments.
(b) How would you distinguish them?

31. A 25-year-old woman gave birth to a baby with haemolytic disease of the newborn which required blood transfusion. She had had no previous pregnancies, had been otherwise well and was on no medication.
Mother: Hb 11.5 g/dl, MCV 80 fl, platelets 215 × 10⁹/l, WCC 10.2 × 10⁹/l (neutrophils 7, lymphocytes 2.5). Group O, RhD positive (*CDe/CDe*).
Father: Group O, RhD negative (*cde/cde*).
Baby: Hb 8.6 g/dl, MCV 102 fl, platelets 196 × 10⁹/l, WCC 14 × 10⁹/l (neutrophils 7, lymphocytes 7). Blood film

showed polychromasia. Group O, RhD positive (*Cde/cde*).
Coombs' test: positive (IgG).

(a) What is the most likely cause of the haemolytic
anaemia?
(b) What are the implications for further pregnancies?

32. A 19-year-old woman presented to her general practitioner
with tiredness and fatigue. She had no other specific
complaints, other than heavy periods which had not been
helped by the use of the oral contraceptive. She had had no
major illnesses or operations and was on no medication. She
was a college student living with her parents. She had a
good diet consisting of meat and vegetables.
Hb 8.9 g/dl, MCV 67 fl, MCHC 31 g/dl, red cell
distribution width (RDW) 21%, platelets 579 × 10⁹/l, WCC
6.7 × 10⁹/l (neutrophils 5.1, lymphocytes 1.4). PT 15 s
(control 15 s), APTT 47 s (control 38 s), fibrinogen 4.0 g/l.

(a) What sort of anaemia has this woman developed, and
what is the most likely reason?
(b) Give 3 essential tests to substantiate your answer to (a).

33. A 17-year-old boy had a sore throat for 3 days and his
general practitioner prescribed aspirin gargles. He returned
1 week later with lymphadenopathy and a persisting sore
throat, but he also felt profoundly tired. He was mildly
icteric.
Hb 8.6 g/dl, MCV 96 fl, platelets 168 × 10⁹/l, WCC 8.1 ×
10⁹/l (neutrophils 0.9, lymphocytes 6.3). Blood film showed
polychromasia with some agglutinates, and many reactive
lymphocytes. Coombs' test positive (complement).
Reticulocytes 216 × 10⁹/l.

(a) Summarize the haematological pathology.
(b) What is the most likely cause and how would you
confirm this?
(c) What treatment may help?

34. A 54-year-old woman had been treated for rheumatoid

disease for 5 years. She had received a number of NSAIDs and a course of D-penicillamine previously. Her disease was considered quiescent and affected mainly her hands and elbows; she had no nodules. Erosions were seen in radiographs of the hands. She was a housewife. She did not smoke or drink. She lived with her husband. She had had 3 normal pregnancies. She admitted to no other specific systemic complaints.

Hb 8.6 g/dl, MCV 91 fl, platelets 203 × 10⁹/l, WCC 6.9 × 10⁹/l (neutrophils 4.1, lymphocytes 2.0). Blood film showed normochromic anaemia with occasional Pappenheimer inclusions. Serum ferritin 200 μg/l, folate 3 μg/l, B$_{12}$ 314 ng/l. Serum iron 16 mmol/l, total iron binding capacity (TIBC) 57 mmol/l, % saturation 30%. Serum sodium 139 mmol/l, potassium 4.5 mmol/l, urea 6.3 mmol/l, creatinine 113 μmol/l, calcium 2.46 mmol/l, AST 47 U/l, Alk Phos 125 u/l.

(a) Give 2 possible causes for her anaemia.
(b) How would you distinguish them?

35. A 55-year-old man with myasthenia gravis and thymoma had been receiving pyridostigmine bromide (Mestinon) for 8 months with some improvement. However, he became more tired and dyspnoeic. On examination, his myasthenia was well controlled but he appeared pale.

Hb 7.9 g/dl, MCV 94 fl, platelets 276 × 10⁹/l, WCC 8.9 × 10⁹/l (neutrophils 6, lymphocytes 2.2). Reticulocytes 79 × 10⁹/l. Blood film showed normochromic features, no fragmentation. Serum sodium 142 mmol/l, potassium 4.7 mmol/l, urea 5.7 mmol/l, creatinine 112 μmol/l, calcium 2.34 mmol/l, albumin 39 g/l, globulin 25 g/l, AST 41 U/l, Alk Phos 106 U/l.

(a) What is the most likely cause for the anaemia?
(b) How would this be confirmed?
(c) What treatment would you suggest?

36. A 76-year-old man presented with tiredness to his general practitioner. He was a retired factory worker. He smoked 10 cigarettes per day and consumed 10 units of alcohol per

week. He was on no medication. Examination was
essentially normal except for pallor.
Hb 9.2 g/dl, MCV 96 fl, platelets 36 × 10⁹/l, WCC 10.7
(rejected differential). Blood film showed polychromasia,
poikilocytosis and fragmentation with an occasional
nucleated red cell and myelocyte. Bone marrow aspirate was
dry. PT 20 s (control 15 s), APTT 49 s (control 37 s),
fibrinogen 0.9 g/l.

(a) What haematological diagnosis would you suggest?
(b) How could this be confirmed?
(c) What is the probable underlying cause?

37. A 4-year-old boy with troublesome eczema was referred
because he had recurrent infections and bruising. He
seemed prone to viral infections and had a lot of upper
respiratory tract infections. Clinical examination was
normal except for several bruises on both legs. He had no
siblings and both parents were healthy.
Hb 14.6 g/dl, MCV 89 fl, platelets 15 × 10⁹/l, WCC
4.7 × 10⁹/l (neutrophils 3.7, lymphocytes 0.9). Serum
sodium 139 mmol/l, potassium 4.1 mmol/l, urea 4.2 mmol/l,
creatinine 87 μmol/l, calcium 2.5 mmol/l, AST 32 U/l,
albumin 37 g/l, globulin 14 g/l. Bone marrow showed
plentiful megakaryocytes and normal erythroid and
myeloid activity. A diagnosis of ITP was made, but the
thrombocytopenia was unresponsive to steroids.

(a) Give the most likely diagnosis and a differential
diagnosis.
(b) What is the best management option?

38. A 26-year-old man attended the Sickle Clinic for diagnosis
and counselling. He had no significant history of sickling
himself although his sister had died of a stroke as a teenager.
He was West African by extraction.
Hb 9.6 g/dl, MCV 72 fl, platelets 220 × 10⁹/l, WCC 6.7 ×
10⁹/l (neutrophils 4.2, lymphocytes 2). Sickledex positive.
Cellulose acetate electrophoresis (pH 7.9): Hb S 62%, Hb F
9%, Hb A 24%, Hb A₂ 5%.

(a) What is the most likely diagnosis?
(b) What advice would you give regarding surgery and family planning?

39. A 34-year-old mother of 2 reattended the Haematology Unit with increasing dyspnoea. She had been treated for Hodgkin's disease 10 years before with radiotherapy and chemotherapy (mustine, anthracycline, vincristine, prednisolone, procarbazine). Examination revealed pulse 110/min (sinus rhythm), BP 130/80. There were some crepitations at both bases. There was no lymphadenopathy or hepatosplenomegaly.
CXR showed a large heart with possible shadowing at the right base. CT scan showed no evidence of recurrent Hodgkins's disease. V/Q scan was normal.
Hb 14.5 g/dl, WCC 8.4 × 10⁹/l (neutrophils 5.3, lymphocytes 2.5), platelets 397 × 10⁹/l. Serum urea and electrolytes normal. AST 36 U/l, GGT 37 U/l.

(a) What is the most likely diagnosis?
(b) What further investigations are required?

40. A 45-year-old diabetic man had been receiving haemodialysis for 2 years. Hb 6.5 g/l, MCV 78 fl, WCC 6.4 × 10⁹/l (neutrophils 3.2, lymphocytes 2.7), platelets 93 × 10⁹/l. He was commenced on epoetin at 2000 IU s.c. twice weekly. This was increased to 4000 IU twice weekly, but the Hb did not improve.

(a) What is the most likely reason for this unresponsiveness?
(b) Give a differential diagnosis.

DATA INTERPRETATION
ANSWERS

1. (a) Hereditary spherocytosis. Note the high MCHC due to the high haemoglobin concentration in the small but densely packed spherocytes. The reticulocyte count suggests ongoing haemolysis, but the negative Coombs' test points away from an autoimmune cause.
   (b) Blood film, osmotic fragility, glycerol lysis time.
   (c) Folic acid to avoid rapid depletion of folate stores. No other definitive action is required and splenectomy is best avoided in pregnancy.

2. (a) Antithrombin III deficiency; ATIII assay. This disorder often causes thrombosis in unusual sites. Because heparin mediates its effect through ATIII, heparinization can be a problem. These two clues point away from the other causes of thrombophilia.
   (b) Protein S deficiency (protein S assay), protein C deficiency (protein C assay).
   Lupus anticoagulant (DRVVT).
   Plasminogen deficiency (plasminogen assay).
   Plasminogen activator inhibitor-1 (PAI-1) deficiency (PAI-1 assay).

3. (a) Paroxysmal nocturnal haemoglobinuria (PNH). This can present with thrombosis, haemolysis and/or marrow hypoplasia. This case is predominantly haemolytic, but there is a degree of cytopenia as well, in spite of a normocellular marrow. PNH has many clinical guises and is not always associated with morning haemoglobinuria.
   (b) Ham's test. Sucrose lysis test. These tests optimize complement activity – PNH erythrocytes do not

withstand this type of stress very readily (they lack the molecules that normally protect against complement-activated cell lysis). As a consequence, haemolysis results.

4. (a) Heparin-induced thrombocytopenia. This is not that uncommon, and may be relatively mild. Several mechanisms have been put forward, including heparin/heparin antibody complexes binding to platelets. More severe cases may result in bleeding or a thrombotic tendency related to platelet clumping.

   (b) Platelet aggregation tests performed in the presence of heparin ± patient's plasma. In this situation, no agonist (such as ADP or ristocetin) is required because the heparin/antibody complex stimulates aggregation, although heparin and antibody do not cause aggregation on their own. Alternatively, platelets radiolabelled with serotonin will release radioactivity in the presence of heparin plus patient's plasma, but again not in the presence of heparin or antibody alone.

   (c) Stop heparin. Prostacyclin is an alternative to heparin in the haemodialysis situation.

5. (a) Acquired haemophilia (autoantibody to factor VIII). Acquired VIII inhibitors can occur in malignancy, autoimmune disorders, drugs (e.g. penicillin), or idiopathically. This can often cause painful muscle and subcutaneous bleeds; joint bleeding is uncommon (compare inherited haemophilia).

   (b) Factor VIII levels are often less than 1% of normal. Factor VIII inhibitor assay (Bethesda assay).

6. (a) Erythrocyte agglutination and haemolysis due to cold antibody production in association with mycoplasma infection. The raised MCV and MCHC is an artefact due to erythrocyte clumping during analysis by the automated cell counter.

   (b) Cold antibodies (polyclonal) or 'agglutinins' with specificity for the I antigen on the erythrocyte surface.

(c) If transfusion is required this should be performed very carefully using warmed blood and keeping the patient in a warm room. Steroids and plasmapheresis are of little use.

7. (a) Chronic myeloid leukaemia with cerebral leukostasis. This is nearly always associated with a poor prognosis. A leukaemoid reaction secondary to neurological infection is a possibility, but the 2-week prodrome suggests a more slowly progressive pathology. Furthermore, the differential is too left-sided for a leukaemoid reaction, and thrombocytosis is commonly a feature of CML.

(b) A leukocyte alkaline phosphatase (LAP or NAP) score can be performed on a blood film in about 1 hour (Philadelphia karyotyping takes days). Typically the LAP score is low in CML but normal/raised in infective leukocytosis.

(c) In addition to hydration, leukapharesis should be considered. Although this *can* give dramatic results, the procedure only produces a small reduction in the WCC which soon climbs back to the untreated level. Intravenous anthracycline will bring the WCC down in a matter of days.

8. (a) Chronic lymphocytic leukaemia; reticulocytosis and polychromasia suggests haemolysis. Lymphocyte surface markers typically reveal CD5 and CD19 positivity.

(b) Haemolysis – Coombs' test.
'Marrow failure' due to CLL infiltration – marrow aspirate/trephine.
Folate deficiency secondary to haemic malignancy – red cell folate levels.
Marrow suppression following chemotherapy for the CLL (not in this case) – marrow aspirate.

9. (a) HIV-related thrombocytopenia. This occurs in up to one-third of HIV patients. It may be profound, causing

symptoms, or quite mild. It does not provide an
indication of prognosis or disease activity. It is nearly
always immune mediated and *platelet-associated
immunoglobulins* are usually positive. Institution of
AZT therapy may help; alternatively, steroids and
splenectomy may also help.
(b) Marrow suppression by AZT or co-trimoxazole
(Septrin).
Development of non-Hodgkin's lymphoma.

10. (a) Haemolytic transfusion reaction (delayed). It is
important to specify haemolytic as most transfusion
reactions are secondary to antigens on the leukocyte or
platelet surface. There was no apparent mismatch in
ABO or Rhesus phenotype, and laboratory error is
extremely unusual as a cause of reaction
(misidentification of the patient or sample being far
more common). In this case the patient had no
detectable antibody on serum screening, but the
transfusion stimulated a low-level anti-Kidd (anti-Jk[a])
antibody that she had developed during pregnancy. This
resulted in increasing haemolysis of the transfused
blood as the antibody level rose, hence the haemolysis
was delayed rather than immediate. Anti-Kidd
antibodies can be difficult to detect not only because of
their nature but also due to this tendency to fall below
detectable levels with time.
(b) Coombs' test on patient's blood.
Cross-match patient's serum from before and after
transfusion with donor blood.
Screen patient's serum from before and after transfusion
for alloantibodies, e.g. anti-Jk[a].

11. (a) Iron deficiency with β-thalassaemia trait. The patient is
iron deficient as a result of previous pregnancies. This was
confirmed by a raised zinc protoporphyrin – in the
presence of iron deficiency, free protoporphyrin binds to
zinc and the ZPP goes up. This test provides a 'same-day'
assessment of iron status. However, the MCV is markedly

depressed given the Hb, and the RCC is elevated; these results are more in keeping with β-thalassaemia trait rather than straightforward iron deficiency. It is often difficult to distinguish the two conditions on the FBC, in general, β-thalassaemia trait has a normal MCHC and RDW, and iron deficiency has a raised RDW and a lower MCHC. The blood film does not always provide much help in distinguishing the two. In Asians, β-thalassaemia is much more common than α-thalassaemia.

(b) Serum ferritin, Hb electrophoresis (Hb A$_2$ raised in β-thalassaemia trait). The husband and family should be screened for β-thalassaemia.

12. (a) Acute ethanol poisoning associated with thrombocytopenia. Patients with dypsomania often have thrombocytopenia, which can be very severe; this responds to abstinence. Although there is a background of chronic alcoholic liver disease, there is no evidence for hypersplenism as a cause for the thrombocytopenia (note, no other cytopenias). Furthermore, chronic liver disease does not usually cause thrombocytopenia of this severity.

(b) Blood alcohol level.

(c) A marrow examination would exclude other causes of thrombocytopenia, e.g. acute leukaemia, and may provide definitive evidence of alcohol-related thrombocytopenia (vacuolated and suppressed megakaryocytopoiesis).

13. (a) Post-transfusion graft versus host disease (GVHD). The features are fever, hepatitis, rash, pancytopenia and diarrhoea. There is insufficient evidence to suggest DIC or TTP. There was no evidence of a viral hepatitis or bacterial sepsis. Although this type of GVHD is uncommon, it should be considered in any patient with malignancy. Methyl prednisolone was indicated.

(b) Skin biopsy, which revealed epidermal necrosis with lymphocytic infiltration (CD8+), confirming post-transfusion GVHD. Analysis of lymphocytes in blood and skin for DNA microsatellite polymorphisms would have revealed the presence of (blood) donor lymphocytes, and this could have been confirmed by repeating the donor sample. In most situations like this, only host lymphocytes should be present.

Wang, L. *et al.* (1994) *New England Journal of Medicine*, **330:** 398–401.

14. (a) Benign intracranial hypertension following steroid withdrawal. Cerebrospinal fluid pressure was found to be 30 cm of water (following a normal CT scan of the brain!). Hodgkin's disease is extremely unusual in the CNS, whereas NHL may present in this site.
    (b) Recommence prednisolone and gradually reduce the dose. Twice weekly lumbar puncture may also help to reduce the pressure. Anticonvulsants should be commenced in the short term, with advice about not driving.

15. (a) Further pulmonary embolus due to inadequate anticoagulation. During the first 48 hours of warfarin therapy, protein C may drop more rapidly than some of the other vitamin K-dependent clotting factors, producing a relatively prothrombotic state.
    (b) Overlapping heparin therapy with warfarin for 3–5 days will protect against relative protein C deficiency.

British Society for Haematology (1993) 'British Society for Haematology guidelines on thrombosis in pregnancy', *Journal of Clinical Pathology*, **46:** 489–96.

16. (a) Waldenström's macroglobulinaemia. Confirm by node and marrow biopsy; immunoelectrophoresis to identify an IgM monoclonal protein.
    (b) Chlorambucil in the first instance. Plasmapharesis should be considered if plasma viscosity is very high.

17. (a) Evan's syndrome – immune haemolysis and thrombocytopenia. The mechanism is not clearly understood, but may relate to the fact that red cells and platelets share certain antigens (e.g. Rhesus), which may react with the same antibody.
    (b) Steroids for both haemolysis and thrombocytopenia.

Bone marrow should also be aspirated to exclude other
causes of thrombocytopenia.

18. (a) The patient is probably deficient in IgA. When such
individuals are transfused with blood containing IgA,
severe reactions may occur. IgA deficiency is associated
with autoimmunity and antibodies to food proteins.
The patient should be examined for anti-IgA. There is a
thrombocytosis secondary to trauma.

(b) Avoid further transfusion if possible. If absolutely
necessary, use blood from IgA deficient donors or
plasma reduced normal blood under steroid and Piriton
cover.

19. (a) Hyperviscosity syndrome associated with relapse of
myeloma. This is most common in IgA and IgG3 types
of myeloma. Hyperviscosity can cause spinal
ischaemia/thrombosis (as in this case), heart failure and
renal failure.

(b) Plasma viscosity. Protein electrophoresis would confirm
that the monoclonal band had reappeared.

(c) Spinal cord compression due to myeloma deposit or
vertebral collapse. Cervical spondolysthesis.

20. (a) Hairy cell leukaemia (HCL) is the most likely diagnosis
based on the pancytopenia, splenomegaly,
monocytopenia, dry marrow aspirate and odd lymphoid
cells in the blood. Acute leukaemia is unlikely as few
blasts were seen. Aplasia is unlikely because the
trephine roll yielded cells. No myelodysplastic features
were commented upon and splenomegaly is not
common in MDS. The gangrenous finger was associated
with an infected finger pulp in a neutropenic individual
(vasculitis may sometimes be seen in HCL). It would be
unusual for such an infection to *cause* such cytopenias
and splenomegaly in an otherwise haematogically
normal individual.

(b) Treatment of HCL with splenectomy has become
unfashionable. IFN or deoxycoformycin should be

used, with or without G-CSF to encourage myeloid regeneration. Broad-spectrum antibiotics should be prescribed to cover the infection.

21. (a) Late-onset, or common variable hypogammaglobulinaemia with recurrent chest and intestinal infection resulting in malabsorption. This is an acquired disorder and results in all immunoglobulins being depressed and reduced numbers and function of B lymphocytes.
    (b) Serum folate, B_{12}, and iron. Xylose tolerance test. ^{14}C breath test.
    (c) Monthly intravenous immunoglobulins. Cyclical antibiotics for prophylaxis.

22. (a) Hypothyroidism producing a macrocytic anaemia. Ring sideroblasts may sometimes be a feature in the marrow. Macronormoblastic refers to large erythroblasts which are commonly associated with macrocytosis of non-megaloblastic origin. Autoimmune diseases may occur in the same patient.
    (b) Serum thyroid stimulating hormone (TSH) and thyroid function tests.

23. (a) Platelet storage pool disease. The haematology and clotting were normal except for the bleeding time; this suggests that there is an intrinsic platelet problem causing the bleeding tendency. This is usually an inherited deficiency of δ-granules within the platelet, but it may be an acquired defect associated with uraemia, leukaemia, Hermansky–Pudlak syndrome, etc.
    (b) Platelet function tests in response to certain agonists are abnormal, and platelet content of adenine nucleotides is low.
    (c) For major or critical surgery (e.g. cataracts) bleeding may be reduced following 1-desamino-8-d-arginine vasopressin (DDAVP) administration. Alternatively, platelet transfusion may help, although this runs the risk of sensitizing the patient to foreign antigens, resulting in less efficient platelet transfusion at a later date.

24. (a) β-Thalassaemia intermedia, a milder form of
β-thalassaemia major. The late presentation of this case
is unusual for β-thalassaemia major, and the
haematology is not right for β-thalassaemia minor. In
the absence of systemic symptoms or features, it is best
to monitor these patients before embarking on a regular
transfusion regime. If splenomegaly progresses,
compounding the anaemia, then splenectomy should be
considered.
β-Thalassaemia intermedia usually occurs when
β-thalassaemia major occurs in a 'mild' form, or in
association with α-thalassaemia or hereditary persistent
Hb F production.

(b) The parents need to be screened for point mutations in
their β-globin genes, because they must both be carriers
to produce a homozygous child. They should then be
given appropriate counselling regarding further
children.

25. (a) Primary proliferative polycythaemia (PPP) with iron
deficiency due to gastrointestinal blood loss. The clue to
this being PPP is the high RCC, leukocytosis and
thrombocytosis; not all PPP patients have
splenomegaly. It is difficult to confirm this with
certainty as the red cell mass will probably be in the
normal range because the patient has 'autovenesected'
himself with blood loss. Serum ferritin and iron will be
low. An LAP score will be high and thus discriminate
the condition from CGL.

(b) It would be inappropriate to give a trial of iron therapy
to see if the RCM became abnormal; the Hb should be
monitored. There has been no real indication to treat the
thrombocytosis as yet, but hydroxyurea or intravenous
^{32}P may be useful if the counts rise further. Gastroscopy
and relevant treatment for the cause of the dyspepsia is
also required. Whether there is an increased incidence of
gastrointestinal blood loss in PPP has been the source of
ongoing debate.

26. (a) Myelodysplastic syndrome (MDS – refractory anaemia with excess blasts) plus monoclonal gammopathy of uncertain significance (MGUS). There are several clues to MDS here – cytopenias, macrocytosis, hypogranular and primitive myeloid elements, ring sideroblasts. Stating that the marrow was myelodysplastic would make the question too easy! Ring sideroblasts can occur in all subgroups of MDS.
MGUS occurs in 3% of over-60s and may have an increased incidence in MDS. However, both disorders are common in the elderly and may be concurrent. Some cases of MGUS go on to develop myeloma, but in this case the patient is on the way to leukaemic transformation first.

(b) Marrow karyotype is often abnormal in MDS and may help demonstrate clonality. Common non-random karyotypic abnormalities include 5q –, monsomy 7 and trisomy 8.

(c) As the patient is not very cytopenic at present, supportive management is sufficient. However, if neutrophils fall to less than $0.5 \times 10^9/1$, prophylactic antibiotics may reduce infections. Similarly, platelet transfusions will be necessary if platelets fall to less than $10 \times 10^9/1$. Once the blast population expands further to around 30% and cytopenias progress, then AML-type therapy should be instituted.

27. (a) Sweet's syndrome. A sterile neutrophil infiltrate of the skin may occur in myelodysplasia, myeloproliferative syndromes or other cancers (Cohen *et al.*, 1988). This may reflect abnormal adhesion properties in these neutrophils or may be a response to the presence of cytokines within the skin. The circulating neutrophil count may be normal or raised. The syndrome is not associated with leukaemic transformation.

(b) Most cases of Sweet's syndrome respond to oral prednisolone. Other treatments include indomethacin, dapsone and cyclosporin (Kemmet and Hunter, 1990; Sharpe and Leggat, 1992).

Cohen, P. R., Talpaz, M. and Kurzrock, R. (1988) 'Malignancy associated Sweet's syndrome: a review of the world literature', *Journal of Clinical Oncology*, **6**: 1987–97.

Kemmett, D. and Hunter J. A. A. (1990) 'Sweet's syndrome: a clinicopathologic review of twenty-nine cases', *Journal of the American Academy of Dermatology*, **23**: 503–7.

Sharpe, G. R. and Leggat, H. M. (1992) 'A case of Sweet's syndrome and myelodysplasia. Response to cyclosporin', *British Journal of Dermatology*, **127**: 538–9.

28. (a) Post-transfusion purpura (PTP). Clearly the patient does not have DIC or marrow infiltrations. The timing is just right for PTP.

    (b) PTP occurs when an individual who is negative for a platelet antigen such as human platelet antigen-1 (HPA-1a) is transfused with blood containing platelets that are HPA-1a positive. Antibodies develop which then destroy the patient's own platelets, even though they are HPA-1a negative. In the acute thrombocytopenic phase it is difficult to measure HPA-1a status due to low counts and a mixture of host and donor platelets. However, anti-HPA-1a can be demonstrated in the serum. If an HPA-1a-positive fetus sensitizes an HPA-1a-negative mother, then intrauterine allogeneic thrombocytopenia can ensue with severe consequences.

    (c) Intravenous immunoglobulin usually produces a fairly rapid rise in the platelet count. Steroids are less effective. (Taaning and Svejgaard, 1994). Platelet transfusion would be inappropriate.

Taaning, E. and Svejgaard, A. (1994) 'Post transfusion purpura', *Transfusion Medicine*, **4**: 1–8.

29. (a) Factor IX deficiency (Christmas disease, haemophilia B) is more likely than deficiencies of the other factors involved in the intrinsic system (XL, XII). Deficiencies of factors II, V and X would cause prolonged PT and APTT. Deficiency of factor VII would prolong the PT but not the APTT. The history is wrong for vWD. Christmas disease is less common than haemophilia A, but has a very similar clinical pattern. Like haemophilia A, the clinical severity depends on the degree of factor

deficiency, i.e. < 1% factor IX level almost always results in individuals being severely affected. However, haemophilia B usually results from gene deletion, whereas haemophilia A results from point mutation within the gene.

(b) Factor IX assay. Haemophilia B is inherited as a sex-linked disorder and family studies should be performed looking for carriers. This is now performed by RFLP analysis. The present case will have a particular band(s) on Southern blot analysis when his factor IX gene is enzyme cleaved; if his sisters have a matching band, it is likely that they are carriers. The technique is performed with several enzymes to avoid mistakes and the results have a high degree of accuracy. It is no longer sufficient to assay factor IX in potential carriers as a means of carrier detection.

30. (a) Chronic granulocytic leukaemia (GCL). Myelofibrosis. This pattern is not typical for transformation to acute leukaemia (platelets are nearly always low). Each myeloproliferative syndrome is able to change into a different subgroup of myeloproliferative disease or acute leukaemia. Marrow fibrosis can be a feature of CGL, especially against a background of previous myeloproliferative disease, and this results in a leukoerythroblastic film. Myelofibrosis develops in up to 20% of cases PPP and would also fit this picture, although platelets can be low or high.

(b) CGL – Philadelphia chromosome in marrow and blood cells; low LAP score; marrow trephine may be hypercellular with or without fibrosis.
Myelofibrosis – Philadelphia chromosome negative; LAP score high or normal; marrow trephine fibrotic rather than hypercellular.
It should be noted that myelofibrosis can be a patchy disorder (like myeloma) and a trephine may hit less fibrotic patches.

31. (a) Anti-Rhc has developed in the mother; this has passed across the placenta and caused haemolysis in the baby,

who possesses c on its red cells. The Rhesus system is complicated, but each Rhesus gene complex may possess *C* or *c, E* or *e, D* or *d* (although *d* is equivalent to an absence of *D*). When a mother is exposed to an antigen she does not possess, she has the potential to develop antibodies to this antigen. This situation can arise in RhD-negative women carrying RhD-positive children, or in group O mothers carrying A or B children. The incidence of RhD-related newborn haemolysis is declining due to anti-RhD prophylaxis in RhD-negative women, but it can still cause severe problems. ABO incompatability tends to cause mild self-limiting haemolysis. There remains, therefore, a group of antibodies that can still cause severe haemolysis in the newborn, anti-Rhc is the commonest after anti-RhD. Anti-Rhc can cause problems in the first pregnancy, classically anti-RhD causes increasing problems from the second pregnancy onwards. The anti-Rhc was not picked up by initial antenatal screening because it developed during the pregnancy once the fetus had sensitized the mother.

(b) In future pregnancies, maternal anti-Rhc levels must be monitored regularly. If there are indications that antibody levels are increasing, then fetal blood sampling may be necessary, followed by intrauterine transfusion through the umbilical vein.

32. (a) Iron deficiency anaemia secondary to Von Willebrand's disease (vWD). The blood count showed classical iron deficiency indices (low MCV and MCH, raised RDW) with an attendant secondary thrombocytosis (platelet function is normal in such cases). There was an isolated prolongation of the APTT with normal fibrinogen – the differential diagnosis is vWD, haemophilia A or B carrier, deficiency of factors XI or XII. Carriers for haemophilia usually have a normal or a marginally prolonged APTT and are usually asymptomatic. Factor XI and XII deficiency are very rare. vWD occurs in up to 1% of the population; the majority of cases are

inherited in an autosomal dominant fashion, causing a mild to moderate bleeding tendency (autosomal recessively inherited vWD is much more severe).

(b) Serum ferritin to confirm iron deficiency. Von Willebrand factor antigen (vWFAg) and ristocetin cofactor assay (RiCof). Factor VIII assay alone will not distinguish a haemophilia carrier from vWD. vWFAg is quantified immunometrically. RiCof is measured by suspending normal platelets in patients' plasma, then stimulating platelet aggregation with ristocetin – as this requires vWF, aggregation will not occur in vWD plasma. Protein electrophoresis followed by immunofixation will determine the pattern of vW multimers and help to subtype the vWD. A prolonged bleeding time is seen in vWD but not haemophilias, as vWFAg is required for platelet plug formation whereas the deficiencies in haemophilia A and B occur after platelet plug formation (an abnormal bleeding time is non-specific for vWD).

33. (a) Coombs'-positive haemolytic anaemia with active reticulocytosis. Neutropenia. Atypical lymphocytes. Specificity on the Coombs' test suggests a cold agglutinin causing the agglutinates on the blood film.

(b) Infectious mononucleosis. Monospot test. This would account for all the findings in (a). The cold haemolysis usually occurs 2 – 3 weeks after acute infection. Neutropenia is not uncommon in viral infections. The reactive lymphocytes are T cells battling with Epstein-Barr virus (EBV)-infected B cells.

(c) Prednisolone will improve most cases of haemolysis, although this should be reserved for symptomatic and severe cases. Transfusion should be avoided if possible because the antibody specificity is to the i antigen which is present in healthy cells. If transfusion is deemed necessary, it should be performed through a blood warmer. Both haemolysis and neutropenia is usually self-limiting.

34. (a) Anaemia of chronic disease (ACD). Sideroblastic anaemia (acquired). Patients with rheumatoid disease should always be monitored for iron deficiency as this is readily treatable. Serum ferritin is not always a good guide to iron deficiency in rheumatoid disease as levels rise in inflammatory states – Perls' stain of a marrow aspirate may be the only way of assessing the true iron status. In the present case there is no suggestion of iron deficiency from the indices or the TIBC, these are more in keeping with ACD. However, Pappenhemier inclusions suggest an abnormality in iron metabolism and suggest sideroblastic anaemia.

 (b) Perls' stain of marrow aspirate to look for ring sideroblasts. Although much research has been performed on ACD, there are no diagnostic tests: the Perls' stain shows iron in the particles but little in the erythrocyte precursors ('iron block'). There are several hypotheses regarding the origin of ACD: erythropoietin insufficiency or resistance, IL-1 excess, etc.

35. (a) Pure red cell aplasia associated with thymoma, a recognized complication. There are no associations of Mestinon with anaemia.

 (b) Bone marrow aspiration would show profound suppression of the erythroid series with a relatively normal myeloid and megakaryocytic series.

 (c) Prednisolone (with or without azathioprine) often helps. Alternatively cyclosporin, antilymphocyte globulin and vincristine may be tried.

36. (a) Leukoerythroblastic film with microangiopathic haemolytic anaemia (MAHA). Disseminated intravascular coagulation. The poikilocytosis, nucleated red cells and myelocytes are suggestive of a leukoerythroblastic film. The erythrocyte fragmentation and polychromasia suggests MAHA. The prolonged clotting times plus mild thrombocytopenia suggests DIC. These are features of marrow infiltration with cancer plus DIC.

(b) Bone marrow trephine will often pick up cancers that are missed on aspirate or because of a dry tap. The DIC would be confirmed by elevated D-dimers.

(c) Carcinoma, probably prostate or abdominal.

37. (a) Wiskott–Aldrich syndrome. This is a recessively inherited disorder characterized by thrombocytopenia, eczema and immunological abnormalities (note lymphopenia and low globulins: cellular and humoral immunity). The differential diagnosis of congenitally acquired HIV is possible, although both parents were healthy. Chronic childhood ITP is also possible, but the features of eczema and lymphopenia point to Wiskott–Aldrich syndrome. Antibiotic-related thrombocytopenia is another possibility. The marrow excludes malignant haematological disease. Recent viral infections could also cause thrombocytopenia but the history is of recurrent infection and bruising.

(b) This condition is progressive and is best treated with bone marrow transplantation.

38. (a) Sβ-thalassaemia – co-inheritance of one β-thalassaemia gene and one sickle gene, i.e. a compound heterozygote with no normal β-globulin genes present. This compound heterozygous state can be associated with mild clinical features if the proportion of Hb A is 10 – 30%; however, with Hb A < 5% more severe sickling occurs. In both situations there will be moderate anaemia, but not as low as homozygous sickle disease. The MCV was below normal with target cells (both features not normally present in homogeneous sickle disease). Sickle cells are not usually present on the blood film in compound heterozygotes.

(b) Standard teaching is to transfuse homozygous sicklers prior to elective surgery to attain Hb S < 20%. This is not the practice in sickle trait or mild Sβ-thalassaemia; a carefully administered anaesthetic with attention to oxygenation and hydration is usually safe. Family studies should include screening family members for sickle and thalassaemia. Potential spouses also need to be screened in case severely affected children are produced.

39. (a) Anthracycline-induced cardiomyopathy. Although anthracyclines are more liable to damage the myocardium in the elderly, subclinical damage can occur in younger people. This woman went to cardiac transplantation. It is recommended that a cumulative dose of 450 mg/m^2 is **not** exceeded.
   (b) Echocardiography and cardiac catheterization. Congestive cardiomyopathy was confirmed.

40. (a) Iron deficiency. It is necessary to monitor transferrin saturation and provide iron supplements if it falls to less than 20%. Serum ferritin is not a good indicator of iron stores in uraemia.
   (b) Poor compliance, aluminium toxicity, haemolysis, ongoing inflammation/infection.

   Temple, R. M. (1994) 'Use of epoetin in the management of renal anaemia', *Hospital Update*, March: 165–72.

SLIDE INTERPRETATION

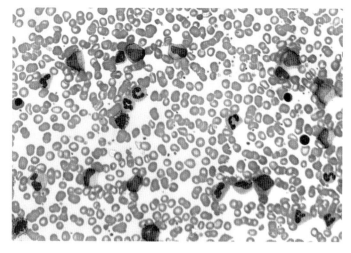

1. This 36-year-old man has had abdominal discomfort and fatigue for 3 weeks. Hb 8.9 g/dl, WCC 87 × 10⁹/l, platelets 655 × 10⁹/l.

   (a) What is the most likely diagnosis?
   (b) How would you confirm this?

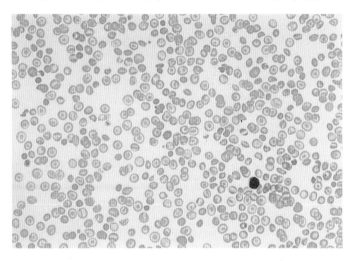

2. This 23-year-old African woman was in her first pregnancy
   and was experiencing increasing dyspnoea. Hb 8.5 g/dl,
   MCV 73 fl, WCC 7.4 × 10⁹/l, platelets 322 × 10⁹/l.

   (a) Describe the main abnormality on the film.
   (b) What is the most likely diagnosis?
   (c) How would you confirm this?

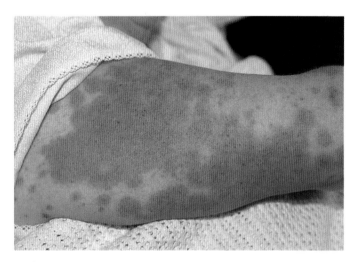

3. This 57-year-old had acute leukaemia. Give 2 possible
   causes for this rash.

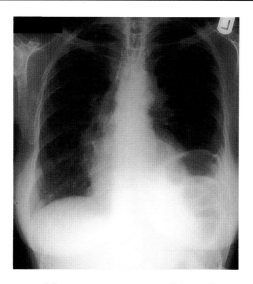

4. This 60-year-old woman was treated for a haematological malignancy. She had experienced increasing dyspnoea of late.

   (a) Describe the abnormalities on the CXR.
   (b) How may these be accounted for?

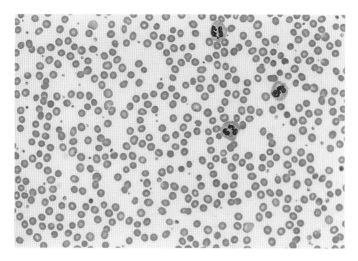

5. This 34-year-old man has a longstanding anaemia. Hb 10.2 g/dl, MCV 83 fl, MCHC 36 g/dl, WCC 12.0×10^9/l, platelets 544×10^9/l.

   (a) What is the diagnosis?
   (b) How would you confirm this?

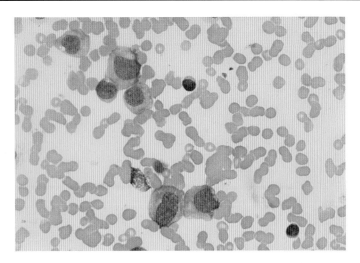

6. This is the blood film from a 34-year-old man who complained of fatigue. Hb 9.8 g/dl, WCC 82 × 10⁹/l, platelets 23 × 10⁹/l.

(a) What is the diagnosis?
(b) How should this be confirmed?

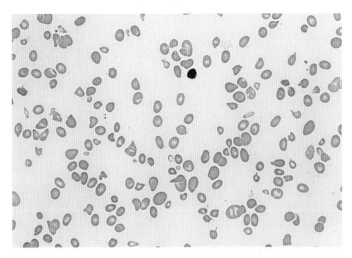

7. This 59-year-old woman had been confused for 1 month. Hb 5.4 g/dl, WCC 2.3 × 10⁹/l (neutrophils 1.0, lymphocytes 1.3), platelets 66 × 10⁹/l. This is her blood film.

(a) Describe the features.
(b) What is the diagnosis?
(c) Give 2 tests to confirm this.

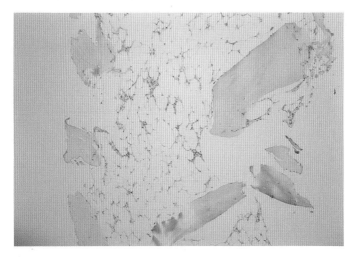

8. This 24-year-old man had difficulty with his vision. Hb 7.8 g/dl, WCC 2.2 × 10⁹/l (neutrophils 0.2, lymphocytes 2), platelets 10 × 10⁹/l.

   (a) What is the most likely diagnosis from this marrow trephine?
   (b) Give 2 features in the history that you would seek.

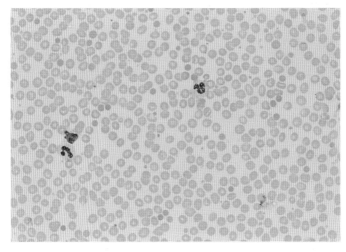

9. What industrial injury has this man sustained? Hb 13.2 g/dl, platelets 566 × 10⁹/l, WCC 15.0 × 10⁹/l (neutrophils 12.5, lymphocytes 2.2).

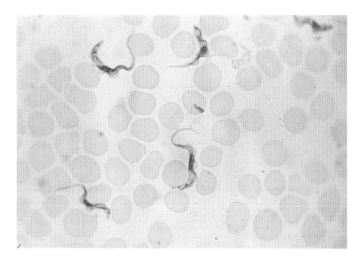

10. (a) What is the diagnosis?
    (b) What treatment is indicated?

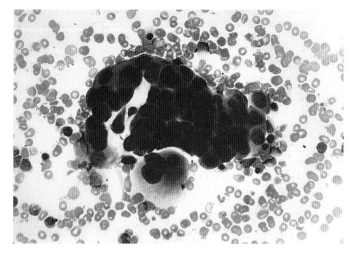

11. A 57-year-old electrician was admitted with pneumonia. Hb
    13.1 g/dl, WCC 15.2 × 10⁹/l (neutrophils 12.1, lymphocytes
    2.6), platelets 47 × 10⁹/l. This is part of the bone marrow
    aspirate that was performed.

    (a) Name 2 features.
    (b) What is the most likely diagnosis?

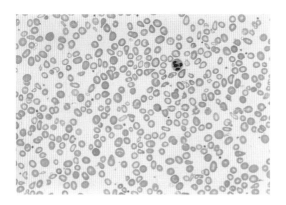

12. This 27-year-old woman had been attending her general
    practitioner complaining of tiredness for 2 months. Hb 11.1
    g/dl, MCV 79 fl, WCC 7.3 × 10⁹/l (neutrophils 5,
    lymphocytes 1.9), platelets 294 × 10⁹/l. She had had 2
    pregnancies and her diet contained meat and vegetables.

    (a) What is the most striking feature of this film?
    (b) Name 2 other features.
    (c) What is the most likely cause?

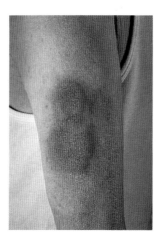

13. This 52-year-old man presented with fever. Hb 10.2 g/dl,
    WBC 54 × 10⁹/l (neutrophils 2.6, lymphocytes 2.2), platelets
    19 × 10⁹/l.

    (a) What is this rash?
    (b) What is the most likely underlying aetiology?

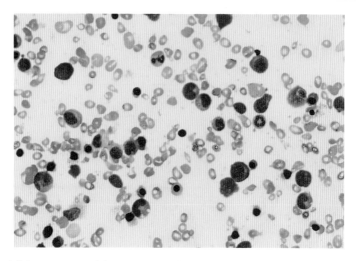

14. This 35-year-old woman with scleroderma became anaemic.

    (a) Describe the main abnormality on her bone marrow.
    (b) What is the most likely underlying cause?

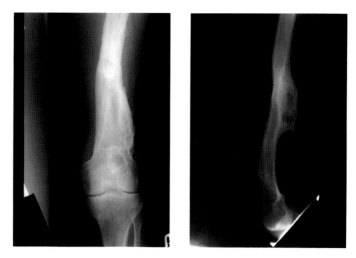

15. This 45-year-old man had suffered with severe Christmas disease. He had had recurrent bleeds in all the main joints. He recently had pain in his lower thigh. What is the diagnosis from the X-ray?

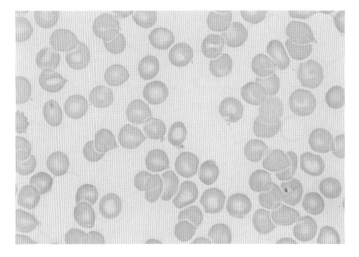

16. This is a high power view of a blood film from a patient undergoing investigation. What is the abnormality?

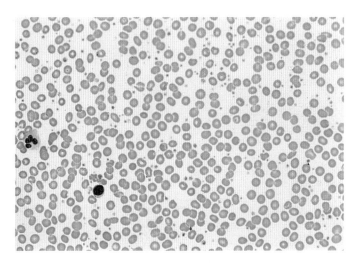

17. This 70-year-old man was admitted with a myocardial infarction.

    (a) What is the principal abnormality on the film?
    (b) How is this related to his admission?

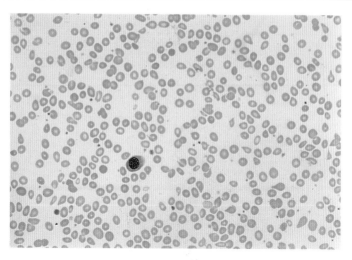

18. This 49-year-old man was admitted with increasing
    tiredness. He was pale and had hepatosplenomegaly but no
    lymphadenopathy. Hb 9.7 g/dl, WCC 13.6 × 10⁹/l
    (neutrophils 9.6, lymphocytes 2), platelets 177 × 10⁹/l.

    (a) Name 2 abnormalities on this blood film.
    (b) What is the most likely diagnosis?

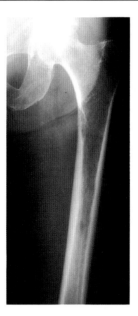

19. This 45-year-old man wanted to go Ten Pin Bowling.

    (a) Name 2 features on the radiograph of his femur.
    (b) What is the most likely diagnosis?
    (c) Would you let him go?

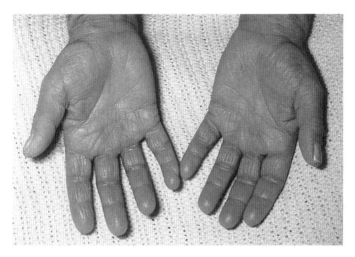

20. This 62-year-old man was under investigation for lymphadenopathy and hepatosplenomegaly.

    (a) Describe the abnormality.
    (b) What is the most likely diagnosis?

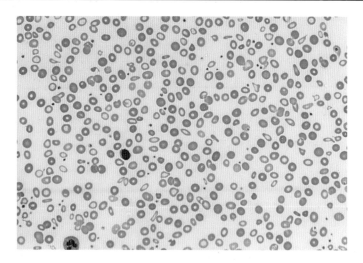

21. This 29-year-old woman had had anaemia since birth. She is Caucasian with no family history of note. She required blood transfusions intermittently. Serum B_{12} and folate: normal. Red cell folate: normal.

   (a) Name the 2 most striking features of this blood film.
   (b) What is the most likely diagnosis?

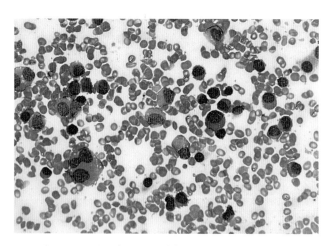

22. This 62-year-old man was under investigation for pancytopenia. Hb 10.3 g/dl, WCC 4.3×10^9/l (neutrophils 2, lymphocytes 2.1), platelet 86×10^9/l.

   (a) Give a diagnosis from this bone marrow aspirate.
   (b) Name 2 other tests that you would perform.

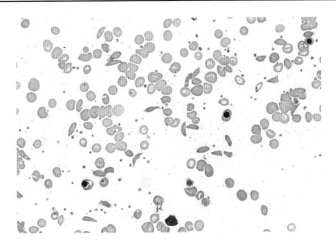

23. This 22-year-old African man was admitted with increasing breathlessness. Hb 6.2 g/dl, MCV 82 fl, WCC 7.6 × 10⁹/l (neutrophils 5, lymphocytes 1.9), platelets 457 × 10⁹/l.

   (a) Name 3 abnormal features from this blood film.
   (b) What is the most likely diagnosis?
   (c) Why has he become increasingly breathless?
   (d) What other complication has he developed.

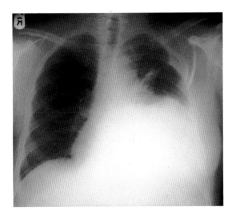

24. This 24-year-old brewery worker went to his general practitioner with increasing breathlessness. He was found to be pale and had lymphadenopathy in the neck. There was no hepatosplenomegaly. Hb 11.7 g/dl, WCC 10.2 × 10⁹/l (neutrophils 7.6, lymphocytes 2.0), platelets 413 × 10⁹/l.

   (a) Name the features on this CXR.
   (b) What is the most likely underlying diagnosis?

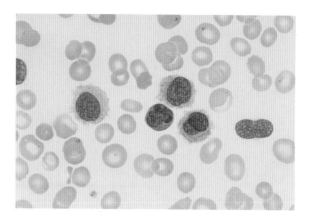

25. This 47-year-old woman is under investigation for pancytopenia. She had splenomegaly but no lymphadenopathy or hepatomegaly. Hb 10.2 g/dl, WCC 5.6 × 10⁹/l (neutrophils 1.6, lymphocytes 2.6), platelets 99 × 10⁹/l. Bone marrow aspirate was unobtainable.

   (a) What is the diagnosis from this blood film?
   (b) What treatment would be appropriate?

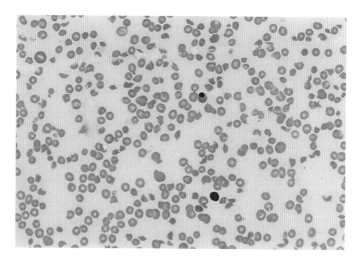

26. This 32-year-old lady was admitted in an unconscious state. She had told her husband that she had felt generally weak and dizzy for the last 2 days. She had recently visited her general practitioner because of urinary symptoms. Hb 9.8 g/dl, WCC 10.2 × 10⁹/l (neutrophils 8.2, lymphocytes 1.9), platelets 8 × 10⁹/l.

(a) Name 4 features of the blood film.
(b) What is the most likely diagnosis?

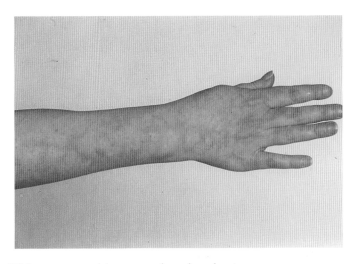

27. This 27-year-old woman has dysphasia.

    (a) Name this rash.
    (b) What is the most likely diagnosis?

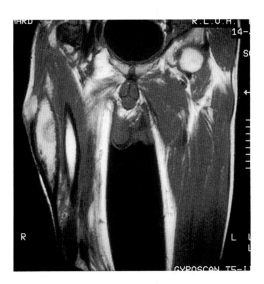

28. This 27-year-old man with severe haemophilia A presented with pain in his right thigh. What is the diagnosis from the CT scan?

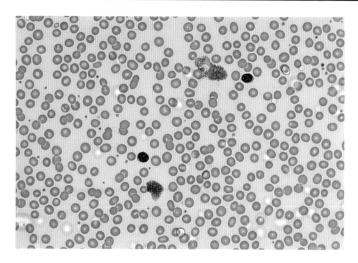

29. This 59-year-old man was admitted for prostatectomy. Preoperative blood count revealed Hb 12.2 g/dl, WCC 16 × 10⁹/l (neutrophils 3.6), platelets 147 × 10⁹/l.

    (a) What is the most likely diagnosis?
    (b) What is your advice regarding surgery?

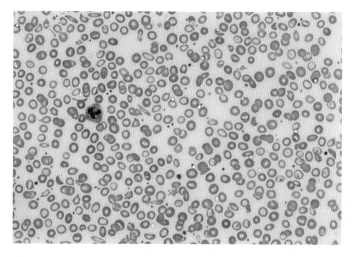

30. This 65-year-old man has been under the cardiologists for many years. He had recently felt tired and was found to be anaemic by his general practitioner and was therefore transfused in the GP treatment unit.
    (a) Name 4 features from this blood film?
    (b) What is the most likely diagnosis and what is its cause?

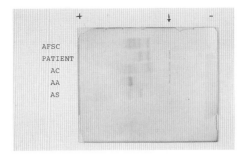

31. This is a cellulose acetate haemoglobin electrophoretic strip. The sample is placed on the gel at the origin (level of the arrow) and a voltage applied as shown. The control lane contains Hb A, F, S and C. The patient is a 27-year-old woman who has had increasing difficulty with her vision.

    (a) What is the most likely diagnosis?
    (b) What other investigation needs to be performed?

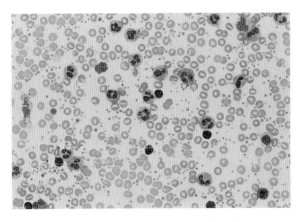

32. This 60-year-old woman was admitted with severe abdominal pain. She had a temperature, was shocked and had peritonism. Hb 10.2 g/dl.

    (a) Comment on the white cell and platelet count from the blood film.
    (b) What is the most likely diagnosis?

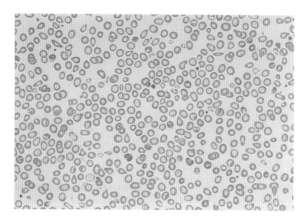

33. This 4-year-old boy had recently moved to the UK with his family, and came to the Haematology Clinic for review. Hb 7.6 g/dl, MCV 64 fl, WCC $6.9 \times 10^9/l$ (neutrophils 3.6, lymphocytes 3), platelets $277 \times 10^9/l$.

   (a) Describe 3 features from the blood film.
   (b) What is the most likely diagnosis?
   (c) How can this be confirmed?

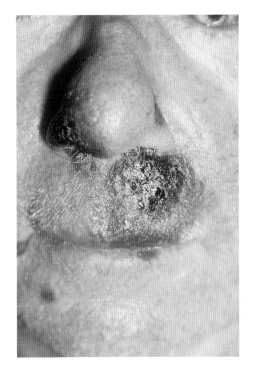

34. This 68-year-old man presented to casualty with increasing visual difficulty in his left eye, and several skin lesions such as this one on his upper lip. Hb 9.7 g/dl, WCC 26 × 10⁹/l (neutrophils 1.1, lymphocytes 2.2), platelets 11 × 10⁹/l.

    (a) Name 2 abnormalities on this photograph.
    (b) What is the most likely underlying diagnosis?

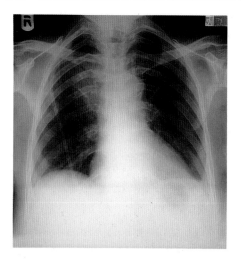

35. This 55-year-old woman has been receiving treatment for acute leukaemia for the last 3 months. She developed a fever with no apparent cause.
    (a) Describe the CXR appearances.
    (b) What is the most likely cause?

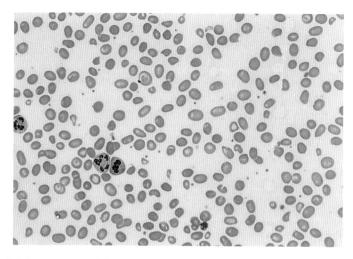

36. This 55-year-old man was seen by the dermatologists for an itchy rash. Hb 7.6 g/dl, WCC 4.3×10^9/l (neutrophils 2.0, lymphocytes 1.9), platelets 112×10^9/l.

    (a) Name 4 features on this blood film.
    (b) What is the most likely diagnosis?

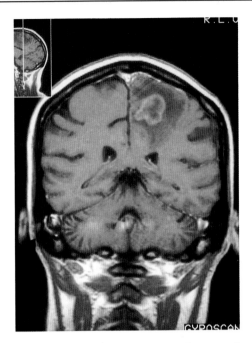

37. This 42-year-old woman had had an allogenic bone marrow transplant for AML. Three weeks following the procedure she developed a fever that did not respond to pipericillin and gentamycin. She had an epileptic fit and was left with a dense left hemiplegia. BP 130/90.
Hb 9.6 g/dl, WCC 2.3 × 10⁹/l(neutrophils 0.5, lymphocytes 1.5), platelets 20 × 10⁹/l. Serum calcium, phosphate and magnesium normal. This is her NMR scan.

(a) What is the most likely diagnosis from the scan?
(b) What is the most likely cause?

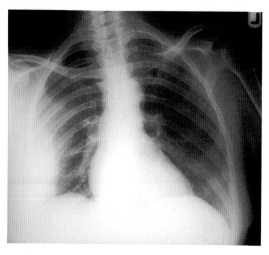

38. This 49-year-old man complained of a dull ache in his right chest. Hb 10.2 g/dl, MCV 89 fl, WCC 7.9 × 10⁹/l (neutrophils 4.3, lymphocytes 2.2), platelets 317 × 10⁹/l. Give a differential diagnosis.

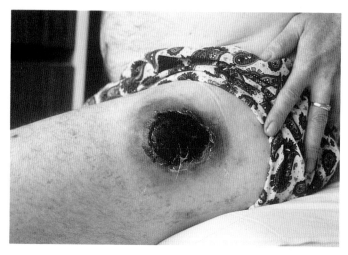

39. This 41-year-old taxi driver presented with tiredness and this lesion on his left thigh. There was no lymphadenopathy or hepatosplenomegaly.
    Hb 11.2 g/dl, WCC 25 × 10⁹/l (left shifted and dysplastic myeloid series, occasional blast seen), platelets 145 × 10⁹/l. Bone marrow aspirate confirmed dysplastic features and 16% myeloblasts.

(a) What is the lesion?
(b) What is the most likely diagnosis?

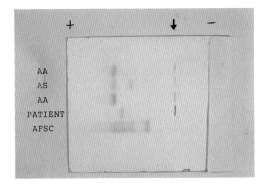

40. This is a cellulose acetate electrophoretic strip from a
    1-year-old Cypriot boy. The origin is indicated by the
    arrow and polarity is as marked.

    (a) What is the principal haemoglobin?
    (b) What is the most likely diagnosis?

SLIDE INTERPRETATION
ANSWERS

1. (a) Chronic granulocytic leukaemia. There is leukocytosis with a marked left shift including myelocytes and promyelocytes. This feature plus thrombocytosis makes CGL the most likely diagnosis. Leukocytosis with severe infection, although left shifted, is not usually as left-shifted as this.
   (b) Bone marrow for Philadelphia chromosome analysis. LAP score on the peripheral blood film.

2. (a) Target cells (also poikilocytosis and anisocytosis, hypochromia).
   (b) Haemoglobin C disease (haemoglobin SC is an alternative).
   (c) Haemoglobin electrophoresis. Cellulose acetate electrophoresis would show a C band running with A_2 and E slightly anodal of the origin.

3. Drug rash (antibiotics, cytotoxics, allopurinol) or Purpura. This rash is not raised and is very unlikely to be leukaemic infiltration.

4. (a) Elevated left diaphragm, deviation of the trachea to the right, possible right lower lobe collapse, borderline hilar lymphadenopathy.
   (b) The mediastinal lymphadenopathy caused phenic nerve paralysis on the left and bronchial obstruction with lower lobe collapse on the right. The patient had non-Hodgkin's lymphoma (NHL).

5. (a) Hereditary spherocytosis with splenectomy. Spherocytes are quite marked in this film and are very

small rounded cells without any central pallor. The high MCHC should also give a clue. Howell-Jolly bodies can be seen and the thrombocytosis gives a clue to splenectomy.

(b) Osmotic fragility, glycerol lysis time, family history.

6. (a) Acute leukaemia (myeloid because of granularity). The large cells with open nuclei and nucleoli which possess lots of cytoplasm are monoblasts. Their size is very large compared to the much smaller mature lymphocytes also seen on the film. The red cell appearance is not true rouleaux, it is merely due to the fact that the photograph was taken from a fairly thick part of the film.

(b) Bone marrow aspirate for morphology, cytochemistry, cell markers and cytogenetics.

7. (a) Gross poikilocytosis and anisocytosis, large oval macrocytes, tear-drop cells, small contracted cells, red cell fragments, thrombocytopenia and neutropenia.

(b) Megaloblastic anaemia. The presence of very large oval macrocytes and such gross poikilocytosis with cytopenias make this the most likely diagnosis. Although there are several tear-drop cells there are no other features of a leukoerythroblastic film. The MCV was not given as this would make the diagnosis too easy. However, in cases of severe poikilocytosis and red cell fragmentation the MCV may be brought back down into the normal range.

(c) Serum B_{12} and folate.

8. (a) Bone marrow cellularity is grossly reduced for a man of 24 years of age, although there are some patches of haemopoiesis. This is the biopsy of aplastic anaemia.

(b) Drug ingestion, e.g. sulphonamides, carbimazole, phenytoin or chloramphenicol. Solvent or benzene exposure. Recent viral illness, e.g. EBV or hepatitis. Family history of blood disorder. Recent cytotoxic or radiation exposure.

9. Burn injury. The presence of very small microspherocytes with the occasional red cell fragment is highly suggestive of this diagnosis.

10. (a) Trypanosomiasis (*T. gambiense*)
    (b) Suramin.

11. (a) Very large clump of carcinoma cells (these cells are much larger than the surrounding haemic cells with darkly staining nuclei and basophilic cytoplasm), megakaryocyte below this clump of cells.
    (b) Metastatic carcinoma, possibly bronchial in view of the pneumonia.

12. (a) Dimorphic blood film.
    (b) Hypochromia, microcytosis, poikilcytosis, anisocytosis, target cells, pencil cells.
    (c) The patient has been started on iron therapy. The dimorphic picture is due to a mixture of erythrocytes made under iron deficiency mixed with much larger erythrocytes which have been manufactured in the presence of iron and which are probably reticulocytes.

13. (a) Leukaemic skin infiltrate.
    (b) Acute monocytic leukaemia. Acute monocytic leukaemias infiltrate the skin far more commonly than other types of AML or ALL. Other complications of actue monocytic leukaemia include neurological involvement, renal failure due to lysosyme release by monoblasts and gum hypertrophy.

14. (a) Erythropoiesis is megaloblastic, the larger erythroblasts demonstrate open chromatin and a 'thrush's breast' appearance. There are also three giant metamyelocytes present.
    (b) Folic deficiency due to scleroderma of the gastrointestinal tract, or B_{12} deficiency associated with intestinal overgrowth due to sclerodermatous intestinal stricture.

15. Pseudotumour of the lower thigh involving the femur. Such pseudotumours can compromise the integrity of bone and lead to fracture.

16. There is a malarial parasite in the lower right hand part of the film. There are no specific red cell features on this high power photograph, beware of over-interpretation. Do not forget to look at the periphery of photographs if you are puzzled.

17. (a) Thrombocytosis. There is a great excess of platelets.
    (b) Thrombocytosis associated with thrombotic myocardial infarction.

18. (a) Tear-drop poikilocytes, nucleated red cell, poikilocytosis.
    (b) Myelofibrosis.

19. (a) Radiolucency within the bone cortex on the medial aspect of the shaft just below the neck. Small rounded radiolucencies are also apparent.
    (b) Multiple myeloma.
    (c) No. The night after the radiograph was taken he rolled over in bed and his leg fractured spontaneously. I was very glad I had not let him go Ten Pin Bowling. He had a 'Bence Jones only' type of myeloma and this is often associated with severe bone disease.

20. (a) Exfoliative erythroderma.
    (b) T cell NHL involving the skin.

21. (a) Dimorphism, hypochromic microcytic population.
    (b) Congenital sideroblastic anaemia. These are the typical appearances on the blood film of this condition; the racial origin makes sickle cell disease highly unlikely and although thalassaemia is a possibility it does not usually give this dimorphic picture (unless transfusion has occurred). There are no features of spherocytosis or enzyme deficiency on the film.

22. (a) Multiple myeloma. There are many myeloma cells some are vacuolated and at least three have multiple nuclei.
    (b) Skeletal survey, serum immunoglobulins plus protein electrophoresis, Bence Jones protein.

23. (a) Sickle cells, nucleated red cells, Howell-Jolly bodies, poikilocytosis.
    (b) Homozygous sickle cell anaemia.
    (c) Development of a chest syndrome.
    (d) Autosplenectomy (Howell-Jolly bodies and thrombocytosis).

24. (a) Left-sided pleural effusion plus pulmonary infiltrate within the left upper zone. The trachea is slightly deviated to the right.
    (b) Lymphoma, probably Hodgkin's rather than non-Hodgkin's, in view of the patient's age.

25. (a) Hairy cell leukaemia. The four central cells are all hairy cells with eccentric nuclei and a large amount of cytoplasm with hairy processes at the periphery.
    (b) Deoxycoformycin, IFN-α or chloroxyadenosine.

26. (a) Red cell fragmentation, polychromasia, nucleated red cells and thrombocytopenia.
    (b) Thrombotic thrombocytopenic purpura.

27. (a) Livido reticularis.
    (b) Antiphospholipid antibody syndrome. The dysphasia was due to a stroke and this, in combination with the distinctive skin rash, makes the diagnosis highly probable.

28. The patient has had a muscle bleed in the right lateral thigh. The scan shows this collection of blood lateral to the femur.

29. (a) Chronic lymphatic leukaemia. The presence of mature lymphocytes and smear cells makes the diagnosis straightforward.
    (b) Proceed with surgery normally.

30. (a) Red cell fragments, hypochromia, pencil cells, macrocytosis, small degree of dimorphism.
    (b) Red cell fragmentation due to heart valve complications resulting in iron deficiency. The degree of dimorphism is due to recent transfusion.

31. (a) Bands form at S and C therefore the patient is a compound heterozygote, i.e. Hb SC.
    (b) Electrophoresis needs to be repeated under acid conditions to make sure that the band running in the S position is indeed S and not Hb D or G. A sickledex may also indicate this.

32. (a) Substantial neutrophil leukocytosis but little in the way of left shift, thrombocytosis.
    (b) Intra-abdominal infection (actually a perforated caecum). This is a leukaemoid reaction and can be differentiated from CGL by the fact that there is not a major shift to the left. The thrombocytosis adds confusion to the diagnosis but in fact was secondary to infection rather than a feature of CGL. A high LAP score rapidly confirmed that this was not CGL.

33. (a) Hypochromia, microcytosis, poikilocytosis, target cells.
    (b) β-Thalassaemia major.
    (c) Haemoglobin electrophoresis demonstrating that nearly all the haemoglobin is Hb F.

34. (a) Pyoderma gangrenosum of the upper lip and severe infection of the left eye.
    (b) Acute myeloid leukaemia. Looking at the WCC the neutrophils and lymphocytes only account for 3.3 × 10^9/l, the rest being blasts. The man had developed a panophthalmitis which resulted in the loss of his left eye. The several lesions were due to pyoderma gangrenosum, which on biopsy showed a mixture of vasculitis and leukaemic cells. The lesions were very sensitive to steroids. In fact the man went into remission following 4 courses of chemotherapy, and when he

relapsed this was heralded by a reappearance of his pyoderma gangrenosum.

35. (a) Patchy infiltrate in the right upper zone.
    (b) This is a typical appearance of a fungal pneumonia such as aspergillosis. Such infections develop following multiple course of broad-spectrum antibiotics.

36. (a) Macrocytosis, large oval macrocytes, poikilocytosis, multi-lobulated neutrophil.
    (b) Megaloblastic anaemia most probably due to folate deficiency secondary to coeliac disease (the itchy rash was dermatitis herpetoiformis).

37. (a) Cerebral abscess. Haemorrhage does not look like this and is usually fatal.
    (b) Aspergilloma. The woman had an asperillus infection of her Hickman line which had embolized to her brain. Such emboli can also produce limb ischaemia.

38. Right-sided pleural deposit could be a feature of carcinoma, lymphoma or myeloma. There are no rib lesions to suggest the latter. Biopsy confirmed NHL. The anaemia was a feature of the NHL.

39. (a) Chloroma. This is a large deposit of leukaemic cells which has occurred outside the marrow.
    (b) From the given data the man has myelodysplasia which seems to be transforming towards acute leukaemia. However, in his case the transformation appeared in the skin rather than the marrow. He made an excellent response to standard AML chemotherapy.

40. (a) Haemoglobin F.
    (b) β-Thalassaemia major.

SHORT CASES
AN APPROACH

1. SPLENOMEGALY

Always look for bruising, lymphadenopathy, splinter haemorrhages and stigmata of liver disease. If there are no clues begin by stating the most likely possibility rather than rarities. If it is not clear what the cause is, approach the differential diagnosis logically.

Differential diagnosis of massive splenomegaly: myelofibrosis (MF), CML, NHL – only mention malaria or kala-azar if there is an obvious tropical connection.

Differential diagnosis of mild to moderate splenomegaly:
- Haematological (malignant): CML, MF, NHL, Hodgkin's disease (HD), CLL, primary polycythaemia, essential thrombocythaemia, ALL (not AML).
- Haematological (benign): haemolytic anaemia.
  1. Intrinsic defects:
  - Congenital: haemoglobinopathy, enzymopathy or membrane defects (e.g. hereditary spherocytosis).
  - Acquired: burns, liver disease, PNH.
  2. Extrinsic defects:
  - Immune: warm vs cold.
  - Infections: malaria, clostridium.
  - Mechanical: cardiac, microangiopathic.
  - Chemicals/drugs: sulphasalazine, Dapsone.
- Infective: infectious mononucleosis, hepatitis, HIV, toxoplasmosis, CMV, SABE, brucella, tuberculosis, trypanosomiasis, schistosomiasis, malaria, kala-azar, histoplasmosis.
- Hepatic: causes of portal hypertension.
- Infiltrative: amyloid, sarcoidosis, Gaucher's disease, Neimann–Pick disease.
- Inflammatory: rheumatoid arthritis, SLE.

2. LYMPHADENOPATHY

Demonstrate to the examiner that you are palpating each area of the neck and each side of the axillary pyramids. If there is localized lymphadenopathy, look for a local site of infection, including mouth, fingers, etc.

Generalized lymphadenopathy:

- Infective:
    - Viral: infectious mononucleosis, CMV, HIV, rubella.
    - Bacterial: salmonella, syphilis, SABE, brucellosis, tuberculosis.
    - Other: toxoplasmosis, histoplasmosis, malaria.
- Neoplastic:
    - Haematological: NHL, HD, CLL, ALL (not AML or CGL).
    - Non-haematological.
- Immune:
    - Drugs: phenytoin, carbimazole.
    - Serum sickness.
- Inflammatory: rheumatoid arthritis, SLE, sarcoidosis.
- Miscellaneous: hyperthyroidism, Addison's disease, berylliosis.
- Gaucher's disease.

3. POLYCYTHAEMIA

Look for plethora, splenomegaly, evidence of thrombotic events, pruritis, hypertension; check blood pressure. If this is not obviously primary polycythaemia, look for cyanosis, congenital heart disease and lung disease, and palpate for hepatic/adrenal/renal swelling; test cerebellar function.

Causes of true polycythaemia:

- Primary proliferative polycythaemia ('rubra vera').
- Secondary:
    - Erythropoietin appropriately elevated: hypoxic lung disease, cyanotic congenital heart disease, high-affinity haemoglobin, methaemoglobin.
    - Erythropoietin inappropriately elevated: renal tumours/cysts/ischaemia, hepatoma, fibroids, cerebellar tumour, phaeochromocytoma.

Causes of relative polycythaemia:
- Gaisböck's.
- Other: diuretics, alcohol, antihypertensives.

4. HAEMOPHILIA

Examine elbows, shoulders and knees, looking for deformity, crepitus and testing range of movement. Look for evidence of nerve or muscle damage. Palpate for pseudotumours. Then search for liver disease.

Look for evidence of HIV: lymphadenopathy, splenomegaly, *Candida*, CMV retinitis, PCP. Kaposi's sarcoma is rare in HIV-positive haemophiliacs.

5. PURPURA

Determine whether the purpura is localized or generalized. Is there a pattern to it?

Platelet causes:
- Reduced production:
  - (a) Marrow infiltration: leukaemia, cancer, myeloma, etc.
  - (b) Marrow hypoplasia: acquired, congenital.
  - (c) Metabolic abnormalities: uraemia, alcohol, B_{12} deficiency.
  - (d) Megakaryocytic abnormalities: myelodysplasia, virus infection.
- Increased destruction:
  - (a) Immune: ITP, post-transfusion purpura, Evan's syndrome, SLE, AIDS, malaria, infectious mononucleosis, lymphoma, drugs.
  - (b) Consumption: DIC, TTP/HUS, prosthetic heart valves, infections (SABE, meningococcus, septicaemia), hypersplenism, massive blood transfusion.
- Platelet function defects:
  - (a) Congenital: Glanzman's, Bernard–Soulier, storage pool defects.

(b) Acquired:
- – Drugs: aspirin, penicillin.
- – Haematological diseases: myeloma, myeloproliferative states, myelodysplasia.
- – Systemic disease: uraemia, liver disease, SLE.

Non-platelet causes:
- Allergic: Henoch-Schönlein.
- Atrophic: senile, scurvy, steroids.
- Mechanical: venous compression, orthostatic.
- Infective: measles, meningococcus, dengue.
- Hereditary: Ehlers–Danlos syndrome, pseudoxanthoma elasticum.
- Miscellaneous: purpura simplex, factitious, fat embolism.

VIVA TOPICS

PROMYELOCYTIC LEUKAEMIA

This subdivision of AML accounts for 10% of adult AML. It has received much interest of late because all-*trans*-retinoic acid (ATRA) can cause differentiation of promyelocytes and the molecular biology of the distinctive chromosomal translocation is becoming clearer.

Patients with M3 AML usually present with pancytopenia and bleeding. Promyelocytes may appear in the blood, but they always constitute the majority of marrow cells. The bleeding tendency results from a combination of (a) thrombocytopenia; (b) DIC resulting from procoagulant release by promyelocytes and (c) fibrinolysis resulting from elastase release from promyelocytes. The bleeding may be exacerbated by chemotherapy as the dying promyelocytes release their toxins. Consequently, death from haemorrhage occurs in 8–47% of M3 patients – generally those with more deranged clotting doing worse. Initiation of chemotherapy is always supported with aggressive FFP/cryoprecipitate/platelet infusion to minimize bleeding. Once these patients attain a complete remission they tend to have a better survival (5-year survival 40%) than other AML subtypes.

The chromosomal translocation (15;17) is found in the majority of M3 patients. Translocation of chromosome 15 material involves the promyelocytic leukaemia (PML) gene, which normally encodes a nuclear protein with a zinc finger motif involved in DNA repair/regulation. Translocation through chromosome 17 involves the retinoic acid receptor RARα). In the presence of retinoic acid, RARα dimerises with another retinoic acid receptor (RXR) to form a heterodimer that binds to certain target genes involved in controlling myeloid differentiation. The protein product of PML–RARα translocation does not perform normally; if transfected into myeloid cell lines, it confers resistance to the differentiating effect that retinoic acid has in these cells. Thus, the PML–RARα protein mutant may be responsible for inhibiting differentation and antagonizing the activity of the normal RARα; the result is a block in differentation and leukaemia.

Trials with oral ATRA in the mid 1980s suggested that promyelocytes could be differentiated into more mature cells, which were then replaced by healthy non-clonal haemopoiesis. This improved the bleeding diathesis, but remnants of the leukaemic clone were still present – this could then be dealt with by conventional chemotherapy. If chemotherapy is not given, promyelocytic relapse occurs within months.

ATRA therapy probably works by causing the normal RAR to be released from the inhibitory effect of the PML/RARα mutant protein, allowing myeloid differentiation to proceed. Why sensitivity to ATRA alone is lost is unclear. The toxicities of ATRA are relatively mild – headache, arthalgia, hypertriglyceridaemia, dry skin, leukocytosis and respiratory distress. The WCC has to be carefully monitored during ATRA therapy.

The use of intravenous heparin in M3 AML has been advocated in the past to improve DIC. This is not standard or common practice and is probably best avoided.

Warrel R. P., Frankel, S. R., Miller, W. H. *et al.* (1993) 'Acute promyelocyctic leukaemia', *New England Journal of Medicine,* **329**: 177– 89.

Zelent, A. (1994) 'Translocation of the RAR locus to the PML locus in acute promyelocytic leukaemia', *British Journal of Haematology,* **86**: 451– 60.

GROWTH FACTOR THERAPY

In the 1960s Professor Metcalf and others demonstrated that human marrow cells could be grown as cell colonies *in vitro* under the influence of supernatants derived from certain cell cultures. Eventually, purification of the factor(s) responsible for such colonies resulted in the term colony-stimulating factor (CSF). There are several CSFs and each is known according to which type of colony it stimulates, e.g. granulocyte-CSF (G-CSF) stimulates the granulocytes lineage. Certain CSFs such as IL-3 and stem cell factor act on more primitive progenitor cells and expand colony-forming act on cells, which in turn will produce differentiated cells. Other molecules such as IL-1 act in synergy with other factors. Once these factors were isolated, recombinant DNA technology allowed large-scale production because it was realised that these factors could limit the damaging effects of chemotherapy on marrow. They also provided excellent research tools.

Initial trials with granulocyte-macrophage-CSF (GM-CSF) showed that this agent stimulated granulocyte and monocyte counts in cancer patients, and also speeded the recovery of neutrophil counts following BMT and chemotherapy. Although shortening the period of neutropenia, it is not clear whether this confers any survival advantage or reduces severe infections. Side-effects, such as pulmonary infiltrates (GM-CSF causes neutrophil margination in the pulmonary vasculature) and bone pain (stimulated and expanded marrow activity results in pain), were noted as fairly regular toxicities.

The use of G-CSF seems to be associated with less toxic reactions. Again, the agent can speed up recovery of neutrophil counts following chemotherapy or BMT, it may confer an advantage in terms of infections, but it is not clear whether there is a survival advantage. It has become routine practice in the USA to commence G-CSF following chemotherapy; this is not widespread practice in Britain. The agent is very expensive and the lack of definite overall survival benefit makes physicians rather reluctant to employ it. Recently G-CSF has been given to expand the number of blood progenitor cells in the circulation. Such cells can then be employed for autologous transplantation following intensive conditioning. The advantage of this procedure is that it avoids using possibly contaminated marrow, and also cell blood counts regenerate faster than with transplantation using marrow cells. This technique may hopefully be developed so that small amounts of blood (50-100 ml) may be sufficient for transplantation.

IL3 has been less well studied than GM-CSF or G-CSF but seems less potent in its ability to improve neutrophil counts, although it can enhance platelet recovery.

The use of such agents in myeloid leukaemias is controversial as they may stimulate the proliferation of myeloblasts. Some workers have employed this property to try and stimulate blast cells into cell cycle and make them more susceptible to chemotherapy. To date, there seems little evidence that these growth factors promote leukaemic growth or relapse.

The use of growth factors to 'kick start' the profound cytopenias of aplastic anaemia has not been generally successful. Perhaps the use of earlier acting agents such as stem cell factor may improve responsiveness.

Another exciting area is the use of negative regulators of cell growth, e.g. MIP 1α. If this is given prior to chemotherapy it can switch off normal haemopoeitic cells and make them more resistant to the toxic effects of chemotherapy i.e. confer protection. Following cytotoxic administration, the normal progenitors can be turned back on by CSFs - the overall effect is to minimize myelotoxicity.

Erythropoietin therapy has been established in the management of ureamic anaemia. However, its use in haematological conditions has been rather disappointing.

IL-2 stimulates T cell growth. It was thought that IL-2 could be used to stimulate host lymphocytes to kill cancer cells. Press coverage highlighted the danger and expense of these trials. Such high-dose trials have ceased because potential benefits were minimal and confined to a minority of patients. However,

IL-2 may have a role in improving immune responsiveness once a tumour has been successfully treated – stimulating the host response to control smaller amounts of residual disease requires much small doses of IL-2. Other strategies have included transfecting the IL-2 gene into lymphocytes derived from the host's tumour then reinjecting these cells. This is highly experimental but has produced a few interesting results.

In conclusion, therapy with growth factors is still expanding and may provide a significant advance in the treatment of human neoplasia.

Galvani D. W and Cawley, J. C. (1992) *Cytokine Therapy*, Cambridge: Cambridge University Press.

Han, Z. C. and Caen, J. P. (1994) 'Cytokines acting on committed haemopoietic progenitors', *Clinical Haematology* 7: 65–70.

PROTHROMBOTIC STATES

There are a number of well-recognized factors predisposing to venous thrombosis: age, pregnancy, malignancy, surgery, trauma, oral contraception, immobility, obesity, untreated polycythaemia, steroids, PNH, sickle cell disease, homocystinuria, lupus anticoagulant, postsplenectomy, DIC, nephrotic syndrome, thrombocytosis (and possibly smoking). Many patients however have no particular predisposing factor(s). There may be a significant family history in up to one-quarter of patients with venous thrombosis, but only a small fraction of such patients will yield definite evidence of an inherited deficiency of a natural anticoagulant such as antithrombin III (AT III), protein C or protein S. Deficiencies in components of the fibrinolytic pathway (plasminogen, PA, PAI-1) probably do not occur by inheritance. Arterial thrombosis can also be associated with well-defined risk factors: hypertension, atherosclerosis, diabetes mellitus, gout, polycythaemia, smoking, obesity, PNH. This review will not deal any further with arterial thrombosis.

Protein C is a vitamin K-dependent factor which is activated when thrombin interacts with thrombomodulin on endothelium. Activated protein C then inhibits activated factors V and VIII. Protein C deficiency is inherited as an autosomal dominant condition, but homozygotes are more severely affected than heterozygotes. Protein C deficiency leads to an increased risk of venous thromboembolism and superficial thrombophlebitis, rarely arterial disease. Thrombosis may occur in younger people, with or without other predisposing factors. Severe or unusual thromboses can occur and tend to be recurrent. Severely affected infants often develop purpura fulminans and massive thromboembolism, which is usually fatal. Certain conditions can lead to an acquired loss of protein

C, e.g. liver disease, DIC, nephrosis, haemodialysis. Not everybody with a deficiency of protein C should receive anticoagulants; these are best reserved for the treatment of thromboembolic events – life-long anticoagulation for patients with more than one event. Warfarin should be instituted cautiously as this drug causes a further fall in protein C and skin necrosis can occur due to superficial skin thrombosis – heparinization should cover the initiation of warfarin for a full 5 days.

Protein S is a vitamin K-dependent cofactor for activated protein C. Deficiency produces similar clinical manifestations as for protein C, although skin necrosis is less frequent. The mode of inheritance is similar to protein C deficiency. Acquired deficiency occurs in liver disease, DIC, SLE and pregnancy. Management of thromboembolism is similar to protein C deficiency.

Antithrombin III (ATIII) inhibits activated serine esterases (e.g. factors IXa, Xa and XIa) by complex formation. Deficiency of ATIII allows clotting to proceed unchecked. The principal clinical manifestation is recurrent venous thromboembolism in young people, often involving unusual sites, with or without a precipitating cause. Arterial thrombosis is less commonly seen. Inheritance is autosomal dominant, in a similar manner to protein C deficiency. Anticoagulation with heparin may prove difficult as this agent requires ATIII for its full effect – 'heparin resistance' may require large doses of heparin followed by warfarinization. Alternatively, ATIII concentrates are now available and may be used in addition to heparin to cover thrombotic events or as prophylaxis in pregnancy. As thromboembolism seems more severe in ATIII deficiency, homozygotes should probably receive anticoagulation for life; indeed, there is a body of thought that suggests that asymptomatic heterozygotes should be anticoagulated prophylactically. Finally, ATIII deficiency may be acquired in liver disease, nephrosis, DIC and asparaginase therapy.

The lupus anticoagulant was so named because plasma from some SLE patients was found to contain an inhibitor (an antiphospholipid antibody) that prolonged the APTT. This antibody binds to platelet phosphoserine and phosphocholine and impairs clotting activation; it also interferes with protein C activation, resulting in a prothrombotic state. Such antibodies are not confined to SLE but can occur in association with pregnancy, hydralazine therapy, phenothiazines, syphilis, HIV, rheumatoid arthritis – thus 'lupus' is inappropriate, the term 'antiphospholipid syndrome' (APS) is more appropriate. A prolonged APTT is insufficient to diagnose lupus anticoagulant activity, a DRVVT is specific because the antibody interferes with the venom activating factor X in the presence of small amounts of platelet material. The antibody can be detected directly by an ELISA technique. The APS is associated with increased venous thromboembolism (sometimes arterial), fetal wastage and thrombocytopenia. Anticoagulation with heparin/warfarin should be employed following a thrombocytopenic event and, according to the severity, may be long term. The management of pregnancy in the presence of APS requires specialist advice – heparin s.c., steroids and aspirin have all been used.

The inherited deficiency syndromes outlined above each account for approximately 3–4% of patients with venous thromboembolism. It is clearly inappropriate to perform assays on all new cases of thromboembolism; however, patients under 45 or patients with unusual venous or arterial thrombosis merit a prothrombotic screen. Similarly, if there are features of APS then this should also be screened for. Such screening should be performed prior to anticoagulation: supply the laboratory with 10 ml of citrated blood for a prothrombotic screen. In addition to a routine clotting profile, this will include DRVVT, protein C and S, ATIII, antiphospholipid antibody ELISA, plasminogen, PA and PAI-1. Once anticoagulation has commenced, performing such a screen on anticoagulated blood makes interpretation difficult.

Creagh, M. D. and Greaves, M. (1991) 'Lupus anticoagulant', *Blood Reviews*, 5: 162–7.
Preston, F. E. and Briek, E. (1993) 'Familial thrombophilia', *Recent Advances in Haematology*, 7: 217–40.

INTERFERON THERAPY

'Interferon activity' was identified when cell supernatants interfered with viral replication. When it was found that IFN could interfere with tumour cell growth, there was a tremendous surge of effort to produce sufficient quantities of the agent for cancer trials. The initial IFN preparation were very impure cytokine soups, recombinant technology has now allowed the production of pure recombinant forms for clinical use (Intron and Roferon). Wellferon is produced from a cell line and is highly purified.

There are three groups of IFN – α, β and γ. IFN-α and -β have very similar characteristics and share the same receptor. There are over 20 subtypes of IFN-α. IFN-γ has rather different properties and has a separate receptor.

Features of the interferons

	IFN-α	IFN-β	IFN-γ
Synonym	Leukocyte	Fibroblast	Immune
Subtypes	Over 20	None	None
Molecular weight (kD)	20	26	17
Cell of origin	Monocyte/ macrophage	Fibroblast/ macrophage	T lymphocyte
Main inducing stimuli	Virus	Virus	Antigen
Effect on human leukocyte antigen expression	Weak	Weak	Strong

IFNs have direct activity within cells by stimulating endonuclease production which degrades RNA – it is apparent, therefore, that IFNs can decrease virus and cellular activity. Many other effects of IFN have been described, e.g. decreased expression of the oncogene c-*myc* leading to cessation of cell growth, inhibition of tubulin and DNA polymerization. In addition to such direct effects on cells, IFNs stimulate immune activity. IFN-α and -β increase NK and cytotoxic T cell activity and improve immunoglobulin synthesis. IFN-γ is a potent stimulator of macrophage activity inducing IL-1 and TNF secretion; IFN-γ also enhances lymphocyte cytotoxicity.

IFN-α is the only IFN that has been used extensively in human studies. Initial enthusiasm led to the use of massive doses with much morbidity, resulting in dose reduction. At the present time, a dose of 3–5 MU subcutaneously each day is much commoner. If it is given in the evening, side-effects coincide with sleep and are then minimized. Fever and 'flu-like' symptoms occur soon after starting IFN-α; these typically improve, younger patients tolerating symptoms better than older patients. Nausea, anorexia and weight loss may become severe and require dose modification. Elderly patients are more prone to develop psychological and neurological sequelae and must be monitored closely. IFN-α suppresses normal marrow function and cytopenias must be monitored. Recombinant IFN-α can induce neutralizing antibodies with consequent loss of clinical efficacy; substitution with Wellferon may overcome this.

IFN-α has enjoyed its greatest success in hairy cell leukaemia (HCL) and chronic granulocytic leukaemia (CGL). Both diseases respond, in 80% of cases resulting in a normalization of the blood count. However, less than 10% of HCL patients have a complete response in the marrow. IFN-α is given for about 12 months in HCL; if the condition relapses on discontinuation of the cytokine, patients usually respond again following reintroduction. Other drugs, e.g. deoxycoformycin, may soon displace IFN as the treatment of choice in HCL.

In CGL, IFN-α can reduce the number of Philadelphia metaphases in the marrow, 10–20% of patients having a complete ablation of the translocation – this represents a substantial improvement on standard forms of treatment and probably confers a survival advantage. The possibility of clearing the disease from the marrow improves the prospects for marrow transplantation and this is still under examination.

The plateau phase of myeloma may be extended by using IFN-α as maintenance following initial chemotherapy. IFN-α is not used alone for disease induction but may be an addition to standard therapies. Whether IFN-α offers any benefit over conventional treatment in low-grade NHL remains to be determined. IFN-α reduces the platelet count in essential thrombocytosis and is an alternative to potentially teratogenic oral chemotherapy. Resistant ITP may also respond to IFN-α therapy – a rebound in the platelet count may be seen following a short course of the agent. It is unlikely that IFN-α has much of a role in the treatment of myelodysplasia or myelofibrosis.

IFN-α can improve lesions of metastatic renal cancer and melanoma – dramatic improvements are not the norm. The other common solid cancers are generally unresponsive to the cytokine. Kaposi's sarcoma can respond well to IFN-α therapy, but with morbidity and uncertainty about whether there is any improvement in overall long-term prospects of HIV patients, the cytokine should only be used within clinical trials.

IFN-α can improve chronic active hepatitis. Patients with hepatitis B antigen may lose this disease marker and improve hepatic histology. Patients with hepatitis C can lose evidence of viral activity and also improve histology. Rhinovirus infection is also reduced with IFN-α therapy, but this can only be justified in immunocompromised individuals.

IFN-γ does not really compete with IFN-α in terms of its effect in tumour trials. However, it may have a place in improving the neutrophil defects of chronic granulomatous disease, and other work suggests that it may modify leishmaniasis and leprosy.

In conclusion, IFN-α has not lived up to its initial promise in terms of clinical benefit. However, it was the agent that opened up the field of therapy with cytokines as biological therapies.

Galvani, D. W., Griffiths, S. D. and Cawley, J. C. (1988) 'Interferon for treatment', *British Medical Journal*, **296**: 1554–6.
Galvani, D. W. and Cawley, J. C. (1992) *Cytokine Therapy*, Cambridge: Cambridge University Press.

MYELODYSPLASTIC STATES

This condition was previously termed 'preleukaemia', an unsatisfactory term giving undue weight to the malignant potential of the marrow – at least half of MDS patients succumb to the effects of cytopenias. It had been recognized for some time that certain anaemic patients would not respond to haematinics, and this could be associated with other cytopenias plus unusual morphological (dysplastic) features in the blood and marrow. The evolution of populations of leukaemic clones within these patients lead to the expressions 'preleukaemia' and 'smouldering acute leukaemia'. In the early 1980s an international group of experts met to discuss the classification of these poorly defined conditions, and the result was the FAB classification of 1982, later expanded in 1985. The term 'myelodysplastic state' was defined as a situation where cytopenias occurred in the presence of a normo- or hypercellular marrow (thus excluding aplasia) with normal haematinic levels. This may arise *de novo* or follow chemotherapy/radiotherapy. The FAB group proposed a classification into the 5 categories given in the table.

Category of sideroblasts	Marrow blasts (%)	Marrow ring sideroblasts
Refractory anaemia (RA) erythroblasts	< 5	Ring sideroblasts < 15% of marrow
RA with ring sideroblasts (RARS) erythroblasts	< 5	Ring sideroblasts > 15% of marrow
RA with excess blasts (RAEB) RAEB in transformation	5–19	Variable
(RAEB-T)	20–29	Variable
Chronic myelomonocytic leukaemia (CMML) – distinguishing feature is > 1 × 10⁹/l monocytes in blood	1–20	Variable

The types of qualitative cellular changes seen are hypogranular neutrophils with abnormal nuclear segmentation, anisopoikilocytosis, macrocytosis, abnormal erythroid nuclear appearance or cytoplasmic vacuolation, giant platelets and bizarre megakaryocyte morphology. The blood features of thrombocytopenia and neutropenia are often features of RA, RARS, RAEB and RAEB-T and circulating blasts may be seen in the latter two conditions. In CMML, the WCC is usually elevated, with dysplastic neutrophils and a persistent monocytosis of less than $1 \times 10^9/l$ ('atypical CML' may appear similar but without a monocytosis). It may seem odd that CMML has been put under the same umbrella of MDS as the other categories, but the marked dysplastic changes and tendency to transform into AML suggested that CMML was biologically a form of MDS. Dyserythropoiesis may manifest as ring sideroblasts in all categories except RA.

The clonal nature of MDS has been demonstrated in a number of ways. Recent work involving X chromosome inactivation with polymorphic markers such as the G6PD, HPRT and PGK genes have been informative in a number of females and reveal that MDS haemopoiesis is usually clonal. In terms of cytogenetics, karyotypic changes occur in 50% of primary MDS and 90% of secondary MDS – trisomy 8, monosomy 7 and deletions of chromosome 5 are commonly found. The presence of such non-random karyotypic changes is strong evidence for abnormal haemopoiesis deriving from a single abnormal progenitor cell, and the appearance of the new karyotypic changes often accompanies leukaemic transformation. Such chromosomal abnormalities may relate to areas of genetic importance for haemopoiesis, e.g. the long arm of chromosome 5 contains the genes for growth factors and their receptors. Other molecular biological studies have shown a high incidence of mutation within the RAS oncogene. The above evidence gives support to the hypothesis that MDS develops, like acute leukaemia, by a number of steps or hits producing genetic instability resulting in loss of control of cell regulation. In secondary MDS there is an obvious initiating event; in primary MDS the initiating event(s) are largely unknown, although benzene and radiation have been implicated.

MDS is quite a common condition in haematological practice and most patients require regular blood product support when symptomatic. Repeated transfusions may require the use of desferrioxamine. Severe infections resulting from neutropenia require broad-spectrum antibiotics and are a major cause of mortality. Although profound thrombocytopenia is not so common, platelet transfusion may be required to reduce bleeding – this situation often leads to platelet refractoriness. If leukaemic transformation does occur, then these patients often prove less responsive to chemotherapy than acute leukaemia arising *de novo*.

The primary acquired form of RARS seen in MDS can be distinguished from the congenital form of RARS on the basis of age of onset (although both have dimorphic blood films, MDS cases have a rather higher MCV). The exclusion of previous TB therapy, lead poisoning, etc., will also suggest that primary acquired RARS, i.e. MDS, is indeed the diagnosis. These diverse causes of ring sideroblasts seem to work through mechanisms disturbing iron metabolism/haem synthesis, the deposition of iron in mitochondria may give rise to free radical formation and consequent protein and lipid damage. Many suggestions have been put forward for the nature of the defects in specific haem-related enzymes, but no unifying hypothesis exists. It is possible that in MDS, abnormal control of proliferation could result in defective protein synthesis and mitochondrial damage.

The classification of MDS into categories assists in giving prognostic information. The survival of patients with higher blast counts and more profound cytopenias is not surprisingly rather worse than patients with RA or RARS. In terms of mortality, death from leukaemic transformation is as common as death from cytopenias, i.e. infection in neutropenia, bleeding in thrombocytopenia. Thus the costs of antibiotics plus supporting patients regularly with blood and platelets makes MDS an expensive condition to manage and much effort has been put into new modalities of treatment.

The majority of MDS patients are over 60–70 years, so treatment is largely supportive with regular transfusions. As there is a high risk of leukaemic transformation, allogeneic marrow transplantation is an option for younger patients (< 45 years of age). Attempts to bring the differentiation process back under control have been made with agents such as vitamins A and D and interferon; these have largely been unsuccessful. Improving cytopenias with growth factors such as erythropoietin and G-CSF can improve counts in some cases; however, care must be taken not to stimulate the leukaemic clone, and cytotoxic agents may be given concomitantly. For patients who have already developed a substantial blast count, AML-like chemotherapy regimens may be helpful if the general state of health is reasonable.

Mufti, G. and Galton, D. (eds) (1993) *The Myelodysplastic States*, London: Longman.

HAEMATOLOGY NORMAL RANGES

Full Blood Count

HB	haemoglobin	male	12.5 – 18.0	g/dl
		female	11.5 – 16.0	g/dl
RBC	red blood cell count	male	4.50 – 6.00	10^{12}/l
		female	3.60 – 5.60	10^{12}/l
HCT	haematocrit or packed cell volume	male	37.0 – 54.0	%
		female	33.0 – 47.0	%
MCV	mean cell volume		80.0 – 100.0	fl
MCH	mean cell haemoglobin		28.0 – 33.0	pg
MCHC	mean cell haemoglobin concentration		33.0 – 36.0	g/dl
RDW	red cell distribution width		11.0 – 15.0	%
PLATELETS			150 – 400	10^9/l
MPV	mean platelet volume		7.0 – 11.0	fl
WBC	white blood cell count		3.5 – 11.0 ×	10^9/l
GRAN	granulocytes/neutrophils		2.0 – 7.5 ×	10^9/l
LYMPH	lymphocytes		1.0 – 3.5 ×	10^9/l
MONO	monocytes		0.2 – 0.8 ×	10^9/l
EOSIN	eosinophils		0.0 – 0.4 ×	10^9/l
BASO	basophils		0.0 – 0.2 ×	10^9/l

RETICS	reticulocytes		4.0 – 140 ×	10^9/l
ESR	erythrocyte sedimentation rate	male	less than 10mm in 1hr	
		female	less than 20mm in 1hr	
PLASMA VISCOSITY			1.50 – 1.72	mpa/sec
HAPTOGLOBINS			100 – 300	mg/dl

SERUM FERRITIN		male	11 – 182	µg/l
	< 50 years	female	5 – 85	µg/l
	> 50 years	female	10 – 93	µg/l
SERUM VIT B12			170 – 590	ng/l
SERUM FOLATE			1.5 – 5.5	µg/l
RED CELL FOLATE			125 – 600	µg/l

PT	prothrombin time	12.5 – 16.5	secs
APPT	activated partial thromboplastin time	26.0 – 33.5	secs
TT	thrombin time	12.0 – 18.0	secs
FIBRINOGEN		1.5 – 4.5	g/l

BIOCHEMISTRY NORMAL RANGES

Sodium	135–145 mmol/l
Potassium	3.5–5.0 mmol/l
Chloride	95–105 mmol/l
Bicarbonate	20–30 mmol/l
Urea	2.5–7 mmol/l
Creatinine	50–130 µmol/l
Calcium	2.20–2.60 mmol/l
Phosphate	0.70–1.40 mmol/l
Alk Phos.	35–125 u/l
Alt	0–35 u/l
Gamma GT	0–50 u/l
Albumin	36–52 g/l
Globulin	22–32 g/l
Bilirubin	2–17 µmol/l

INDEX

abscess, cerebral, 121
acidified glycerol lysis time, 36
acidified sucrose lysis test, 41
acute respiratory distress syndrome (ARDS), 58
alcohol abuse, 57, 75
allopurinol, 115
all-*trans*-retinoic acid (ATRA), 130, 131
anaemia, 93, 98, 102, 106
  aplastic, 25, 116
  of chronic disease, 85
  congenital sideroblastic, 118
  Coombs' positive, 12
  Coombs' positive haemolytic, 39, 84
  Fanconi's, 31
  haemolytic, 21, 22
  hypochromic microcytic, 23
  iron deficiency, 83
  macrocytic, 64
  megaloblastic, 116, 121
  microangiopathic haemolytic, 26, 85
  normochromic normocytic, 14, 19
  pernicious, 62
  sideroblastic, 85
  see also sickle cell disease
anisocytosis, 11, 115, 116, 117
anthracycline, 73
anthracycline-induced cardiomyopathy, 87
anticardiolipin antibody titre, 21
anti-Kidd antibody, 74
antilymphocyte globulin (ALG), 6, 25
antiphospholipid syndrome, 21, 27, 119, 137
antithrombin III, 33, 136
  deficiency, 71, 136
aplastic anaemia, 25, 116
apparent polycythaemia, 34
aspergilloma, 121
aspergillosis, 121

asthma, late-onset, 61
ataxia telangiectasia, 33
atenolol, 3, 10
autohaemolysis, 36
autosplenectomy, 30, 119
azathioprine, 85
azathothymidine (AZT), 55, 74

Bence Jones light chains, 19
'Bence Jones' only myeloma, 19, 118
Bence Jones protein (BJP), 19, 39, 119
benzylpenicillin, 6
biochemistry reference ranges, 146
blind-loop syndrome, 45
Bloom's syndrome, 33
bone marrow transplantation, 25, 32-3, 39
brucella, 124
Budd-Chiari syndrome, 41, 42
burns, 117

C8-binding protein, 41
captopril, 37
carbimazole, 116
carcinoma
  of the colon, 65
  Duke's stage C, 57
  hepatic, 32
  hepatocellular, 49
cephalexin, 57
chlorambucil, 43, 45, 76
chlorambucil/vincristine/procarbazine/prednisolone (CLVPP), 58
chloramphenicol, 116
chloroma, 121
chloroquine, 13, 41
chloroxyadenosine, 119
cholecystitis, 53
Christmas disease, 81, 82, 98
cirrhosis, 48, 49
coeliac disease, 121
colony-stimulating factor (CSF), 132
confusion, 6, 94